D0181756

IIDE TO

MISCARRIAGE & PREGNANCY LOSS

Hope and healing when you're no longer expecting

Kate White, M.D.

OB-GYN and miscarriage survivor

MAYO CLINIC PRESS

MAYO CLINIC PRESS
200 First St. SW
Rochester, MN 55905
http://mcpress.MayoClinic.org

All photographs and illustrations are copyright of Mayo Foundation for Medical Education and Research except for the following:
Cover image: shutterstock_323101352.jpg/CREDIT: © SHUTTERSTOCK
Back cover and page 384/CREDIT: © LORNA STELL PHOTO

The information in this book is true and complete to the best of our knowledge. This book is intended as an informative guide for those wishing to learn more about health issues. It is not intended to replace, countermand or conflict with advice given to you by your own physician. The ultimate decision concerning your care should be made between you and your doctor. Information in this book is offered with no guarantees. The author and publisher disclaim all liability in connection with the use of this publication. The views expressed are the author's personal views, and do not necessarily reflect the policy or position of Mayo Clinic.

To stay informed about Mayo Clinic Press, please subscribe to our free e-newsletter at *http://mcpress.MayoClinic.org* or follow us on social media.

For bulk sales to employers, member groups and health-related companies, contact Mayo Clinic at SpecialSalesMayoBooks@mayo.edu.

Proceeds from the sale of every book benefit important medical education and research at Mayo Clinic.

Managing editor: Stephanie K. Vaughan
Art director: Stewart J. Koski
Cover design: Gunnar T. Soroos
Production designer: Amanda J. Knapp

ISBN 978-1-893005-74-7
Library of Congress Control Number: 2021939040

Printed in the United States of America

ii

For Samantha

Contents

You are not alone

You pee on a stick, you put it on the bathroom counter and you wait.

And you wait.

Those two minutes seem to take forever.

Then finally, you see two lines. And just like that, you're pregnant. You may have waited a long time for this day, or it might have been a surprise. Either way, you know your life is about to change.

Then suddenly, you're no longer pregnant. You may realize when your pregnancy ends. You may start bleeding or have cramping so bad that you know it's not normal. You may suddenly stop feeling nauseous and tired. Or you may have no idea — until you see the concerned look on the ultrasound technician's face after scanning you for a very long time without saying anything.

When you're happy to be pregnant, you don't like to think about the possibility that it might not work out. *Everything will be fine,* you tell yourself. *I'm healthy.* Or, *We tried for this for so long.* Or, *Things have been going well for months now.* Or, *Everyone in my family has healthy pregnancies, so why wouldn't I?*

Miscarriages, especially early pregnancy losses, are much more common than most people realize. Years ago, it wasn't unusual for people to miscarry without ever knowing they were pregnant. The miscarriage would pass — with the person blissfully unaware — in what appeared to be a period, albeit one that was a couple of weeks late. Today, the availability of sensitive home pregnancy tests means that people find out earlier than ever that they're pregnant. And that means that more people than ever know exactly what's happened when they have a late and heavy period, experience out-of-the blue pelvic cramping, or are no longer nauseous or tired.

However, people rarely talk about their pregnancy losses, so you probably don't know that many people in your life have had miscarriages. Chances are that someone in your family has had one that they've never discussed. Multiple people in your social media feed have probably had more than one. No one is immune from the possibility of pregnancy loss, not even your OB-GYN.

I know because it happened to me.

The fact that miscarriage is common makes it no less painful — because it's not common for you. When you lose a pregnancy, you lose more than a baby. You lose your hope for an entire possible future that had sprung into being. It doesn't matter if your miscarriage occurred at six weeks or six months or even later. For many people, it's a crushing disappointment that's felt physically, mentally and emotionally. And the recovery from a pregnancy loss can last longer than the pregnancy itself.

As a gynecologist who specializes in family planning, I've been taking care of women and people who can become pregnant for over 20 years, and the surprises and sorrow of miscarriages leave patients as full of questions as they are of emotion. Even though these appointments last an hour, I know it's often not enough time to talk through everything on my patients' minds. I wrote this book to continue that conversation — to cover all the information people might seek when experiencing a miscarriage, plus the information they will need later but didn't know to ask their doctors for.

It's time we talk about miscarriage. In the United States, this taboo against talking about pregnancy loss has gone on for way too long, as if uttering the word *miscarriage* could cause one to happen. The reluctance to talk about the experience and share our stories has led to too much unnecessary suffering, isolation and misunderstanding.

Maybe you're facing a miscarriage right now and trying to sort through your options. You might have had a loss in the past and aren't sure what exactly happened or why. Perhaps you didn't have any questions at the time of your miscarriage — you just wanted it to be over — but concerns and questions have bubbled up since. Maybe you got this book from someone who cares about you and wants to help but doesn't know what to say.

You may be facing a miscarriage of a pregnancy you're not carrying. Perhaps your surrogate or the birth parent is the one experiencing the physical loss of the pregnancy. This loss is yours as well, but you're not getting assistance from the doctors, and you may be uncertain about how to process your grief.

Or maybe you're not facing a miscarriage. Perhaps miscarriage runs in your family and you want to be prepared. Or your doctor has said you have a medical condition that increases your risk of pregnancy loss. Maybe your best friend or a sibling has experienced miscarriage and you want to be able to help.

In the chapters to come, I talk about the reasons why a miscarriage may have occurred and explore why sometimes the answer is just not knowable. I emphasize the things that don't cause a miscarriage … and why no one should *ever* feel guilty about having one. And I discuss how doctors* figure out for sure that a pregnancy is over, because no one ever wants to make a mistake with a diagnosis like this.

I also discuss treatment. You may be surprised to learn that you have options, and in many cases, you get to make the choice about what happens next. I discuss the timeline of a miscarriage — how long you can expect it to take and how you'll feel at various points throughout it.

I talk about the special circumstances around some miscarriages. Most people having a miscarriage are in the first trimester of pregnancy, but some face losses that are much more medically complex.

Finally, I talk about the aftermath of a miscarriage. I discuss what a typical recovery looks like and when you should follow up with your health care provider. I also help you learn what a miscarriage means for your body, for your heart and for your attempts at trying to get pregnant in the future.

Throughout the book, I share some of my patients' stories (names have been changed), as well as some of the questions and concerns that patients have brought to me over the years. You may be feeling or wondering the same things. I also share my own experiences of miscarriage — a traumatic stillbirth at 29 weeks and a first trimester loss at five weeks. I'll never say, "I understand what you're going through" because everyone experiences loss differently. However, I hope that my story validates your feelings and makes you feel a little less alone.

While this may not be a situation you ever imagined yourself being in, know that having a miscarriage doesn't have to be scary. And it doesn't mean you'll never get to be a parent or have another child. You are *so* not alone — a legion of others, including me, have walked this path before you, and our experiences can guide you along your way. Let's walk together.

*Note: Throughout this book, I use the word doctor *to represent health care providers who may care for you in pregnancy (which includes midwives and nurse practitioners) since physicians are the ones who tend to oversee or perform procedures for miscarriage. And in recognition that not all people who can get pregnant identify as women, I use gender-neutral pronouns whenever I'm not referring to the results of research studies. When talking about pregnancy loss, no one should feel excluded. We're all in the community of grief together.*

PART 1

Preparing

In these first few chapters, you'll learn how someone gets a miscarriage diagnosis, how to interpret the terms that doctors may use, what information you need to help you understand your options for care, and how to get ready for your miscarriage to start.

The first part of this section focuses on general pregnancy loss. Then, this section moves on to first trimester miscarriage, the most common type of loss. You'll find signposts along the way in the book so that you can easily find the information that applies to your individual situation.

CHAPTER 1

Understanding miscarriage: Why did this happen?

Alicia was my last patient of the morning. Throughout her ultrasound, her eyes stayed glued to my face as I searched in vain for good news on the screen. Instead, I showed her what I saw — that her embryo did not have a heartbeat. "I don't understand," she kept repeating. "I'm healthy, I take care of myself. How could this happen?"

For many people, the sudden end of a pregnancy gives rise to a thousand thoughts and feelings. Suddenly, you're not sure what this means about your body or your ability to have a healthy pregnancy, and you certainly aren't sure what might happen next. Of the questions that patients ask me, the first is almost always, "Why did this happen to me?"

A person having a miscarriage joins a club that they never intended to sign up for. This club is full of amazing people from all different walks of life who are bonded together by this similar experience. Everyone's miscarriage journey is different, but you and the others that came before you all experience the physical and emotional loss of a pregnancy ending.

This is a bigger club than you realize. Around 1 in 4 recognized pregnancies ends in a miscarriage — and it may be as many as half the pregnancies, since many people miscarry before they realize they are pregnant. At those rates, about a quarter of women will experience a miscarriage during their lifetimes. This means you absolutely know at least one person who has had a miscarriage, even if no one has told you they've had one.

Miscarriages happen to people in every country and every situation in life. Healthy or sick. Young or old. Happy or sad or unsure about the pregnancy. There are risk factors for miscarriages, but it's important to know that most pregnancy losses happen to completely healthy people.

MISCARRIAGE RISK FACTORS

A risk factor doesn't mean you're destined to have a loss, but it does increase the chances of having another one in the future. Here are the most common risk factors for pregnancy loss.

Who you are:
- **Age.** Being over 35 or having a male partner over 40.
- **Weight.** Being underweight or overweight is associated with miscarriage, but it's unclear if weight itself directly increases the risk.

What you do:
- **Lifestyle factors.** Smoking 10 cigarettes or more a day, drinking alcohol, or using nonprescribed substances, particularly cocaine.
- **Exposure to radiation and toxic substances.** Having a job that exposes you to toxins, like pesticides, heavy metals (lead, mercury, arsenic), solvents (toluene and benzene), ionizing radiation and some chemotherapy agents.
- **Extensive lifting at work.** Regularly lifting over 220 pounds a day. If your job or workplace poses a risk to you during pregnancy, your doctor can write a letter to your employer. Your employer should make accommodations for you.

Pregnancy complications:
- **Multiple gestation.** Twins, triplets, or more.
- **Pregnant with an IUD in place.** Intrauterine devices (IUDs) are highly effective forms of birth control, but if the device fails, the pregnancy is at a higher risk of loss.
- **Invasive pregnancy testing.** Chorionic villus sampling (CVS) and amniocentesis tests to determine if the baby is healthy can uncommonly cause miscarriage.
- **Infections.** Rubella, chickenpox, foodborne infections (listeriosis, salmonellosis).
- **High-velocity trauma,** like a serious motor vehicle accident or major fall; or **low-velocity trauma,** like getting hit in the belly during a low-speed motor vehicle accident in the second or third trimester.

Unclear associations, due to poor or conflicting data:
- **Night shift work.** Some studies (but not all) have shown that working a night shift affects long-term health and increases the risk of miscarriage.
- **Taking medication.** Certain drugs, including oral medication used to treat a yeast infection, may increase early miscarriage risk. Ask your doctor if there are drugs or supplements you shouldn't take while pregnant.

The average person who wants to be pregnant and have more than one child may be pregnant many times in a lifetime. The odds are actually higher that you're going to have at least one miscarriage than that you won't have any. It's especially sad when a miscarriage happens in a first pregnancy because of all the doubts it might raise. But you're no more or less likely to have bad luck on your first pregnancy than your fourth.

IT'S SO COMMON ... BUT NOBODY TALKS ABOUT IT

You might not have known miscarriage is so common because no one really talks about it. For all our share-everything social media culture, a lot of people still aren't comfortable discussing miscarriages because pregnancy loss not only brings up questions about their health, but also about their identities — about their femininity and how well they can do their "job" as women, or if they don't identify as a woman, about what it means for their abilities to parent a child. So, pregnancy loss may be a particularly emotionally loaded subject.

Many doctors may unintentionally contribute to this stigma. Did your doctor tell you, "Don't tell anyone you're pregnant until the end of the first trimester"? Doctors mean well when they offer this advice. They don't want to put you in the uncomfortable position of having to inform your social network that you're no longer pregnant. But keeping a pregnancy secret can lead to feelings of loneliness and isolation. Many people wished they had told their friends and family about the pregnancy sooner, to have more support when the loss happened.

Pregnancies haven't always been kept a secret in the way they often are today. A hundred years ago, before the advent of modern and highly effective birth control, women had many more pregnancies than they do today, so miscarriage was more common. And because care wasn't as advanced as it is today, miscarriage was associated with serious complications.

THE DICE ANALOGY

In medicine, miscarriage is considered an occasional and even expected outcome of a pregnancy. A doctor I know likened it to rolling a die. If you roll a five, you wouldn't be surprised that you rolled a five. You just know that there's a chance when you roll a die that a five could come up. The same is true when you become pregnant. Losing a pregnancy is statistically common — like rolling a five.

Hemorrhages and infections were the norm, and they threatened not only a woman's fertility, but her life. As a result, miscarriages were a more common topic of conversation.

Over time, miscarriage evolved from being considered a common outcome to becoming a public health issue. The 1970s in America saw a rise in activism against environmental hazards thought to be associated with miscarriages. Eventually, as technology and pregnancy care improved, conventional wisdom decreed that every pregnancy should be successful. At that point, most Americans became much more secretive about their miscarriages, as it felt like a pregnancy loss was a breach of expectations, and somehow represented a shameful failure.

CAUSES OF MISCARRIAGES

Why *do* miscarriages happen? Doctors who practice obstetrics sometimes find it amazing that a healthy pregnancy ever occurs, given how easy it is for something to go wrong.

There has not been extensive research on miscarriage, and new information comes out all the time. However, we do know that there are four general categories that explain why pregnancy loss usually happens. Learn more about each category next.

BY ANY OTHER NAME

Doctors may refer to the embryo, the fetus or even the pregnancy. These terms may be medically accurate, but many people also refer to their pregnancy as their baby. Let your medical team know how you want to refer to your pregnancy as the miscarriage is happening. Your medical team should respect your wishes.

(?) YOU MAY BE THINKING ...

It doesn't help when you tell me it's "normal."

In trying to reassure you that you're going to be fine, doctors often stress what a common outcome pregnancy loss is. But, for a person shocked by this news, hearing, "It's normal" can come across as cold and uncaring. Knowing the frequency of pregnancy loss doesn't reduce the impact, doesn't help you and doesn't stop you from feeling devastated. After all, it's not normal for *you*.

Chromosomal

Problems with the embryo's DNA, like an extra copy of a chromosome, cause up to 60% of pregnancy losses. In these cases, the pregnancy wasn't healthy from the start.

One mismatch, or one wrong cell division, and the pregnancy is doomed. Even if the chromosome number is correct, there can be genetic problems *within* the chromosomes that don't allow a pregnancy to progress.

Problems with the uterus

Some people are born with a uterine septum. This wedge of tissue within the womb divides the inside of the uterus into two sections. If the placenta implants on a septum, it can't adequately deliver oxygen and nutrition to a fetus.

A weakened cervix that dilates months before the baby has developed enough to survive outside the womb also can cause miscarriage in the second trimester.

Certain medical conditions

Serious and uncontrolled conditions — like severe diabetes, high blood pressure, blood-clotting disorders, thyroid disease and autoimmune disease — are associated with pregnancy loss. This is because hormone levels outside the standard range, impaired placental blood vessels and antibodies caused by these conditions directly harm the pregnancy.

Infections

Listeria, toxoplasma, rubella, cytomegalovirus, mycoplasma, ureaplasma, chlamydia, herpes virus, parvovirus and a host of other infections have been associated with miscarriage.

WHAT DOES *NOT* CAUSE MISCARRIAGES

Now for a short, but by no means definitive, list of all the things that did *not* cause this pregnancy to be a miscarriage.

Exercise, heavy lifting or physical exertion

Don't worry about the fact that you vacuumed your house, moved a few heavy boxes, or lifted your niece or nephew. Even if you have a job that involves lifting mattresses or pushing heavy carts. Even if you bench-pressed 150 pounds on a few occasions or ran a marathon (which is *amazing*). No amount of typical physical activity can cause a miscarriage.

Working

There's no link between miscarriage and full-time employ-ment, standing more than six hours a day, or an average amount of lifting. While some jobs may be associated with a higher risk (see "Miscarriage risk factors" on page 14), it's unlikely your job had anything to do with your miscarriage.

Screen time

Working at a computer all day or spending a lot of time on your social media accounts is not associated with miscarriage. The electromagnetic fields from computer screens are weak. While staring at a screen all day may not be good for your eyesight or your relationships, it doesn't threaten your pregnancy.

Air travel

Cabin pressurization isn't associated with higher miscarriage risk. However, if you do fly while you're pregnant, be sure to regularly get up and walk the aisle to prevent blood clots in your legs. Pregnancy does increase your risk of those.

Frights

There are myths about a shock or fright causing a miscarriage. That's not true, either. Enjoy all the horror movies you want.

Sex

I don't care how vigorous the sex was, how athletic or in what position. In fact, I hope all those things were superfun. No amount of sex (or an orgasm, with or without intercourse) can disrupt your pregnancy.

Caffeine

Moderate caffeine consumption (2 cups of coffee or 3 to 5 cans of soda a day) is OK while pregnant.

Tampons

Tampons stay in your vagina and go nowhere near the baby inside the uterus.

Hormonal birth control

Hormonal contraception doesn't fundamentally change your ovaries, your eggs or your uterus, and it has no impact on the health of your pregnancies. While the injection can delay your periods from returning for up to a year, you'll still be able to have a healthy pregnancy once the hormonal effects wear off.

If your hormonal birth control failed and you became pregnant while using it, there is no increased risk of miscarriage.

An intrauterine device (IUD)

Similarly, having used an IUD in the past doesn't increase your risk of miscarriage. The only association with an IUD and miscarriage is in the rare instances when you become pregnant *with* an IUD in place. These pregnancies have a high risk of miscarriage, especially if the IUD is not removed.

A past abortion

It isn't uncommon for people to feel that their decisions about past pregnancies are the reason for a present-day miscarriage. Medically, a past abortion — even if you've had more than one — has no impact on your pregnancies in the future. You made the best decision for yourself that you could at the time, and an abortion does not damage your uterus so that you can't get pregnant again. The universe is not sending you a message.

Morning sickness

My patients have asked me if their babies were nutritionally deprived because they were nauseous all the time and couldn't eat or were vomiting throughout the day. No matter how much you vomited or how little you ate, morning sickness does not lead to miscarriage. In fact, it's associated with high pregnancy hormone levels that tend to indicate healthier pregnancies.

A flu shot

The effects of flu vaccines on pregnancies have been heavily researched. Despite what you may have heard, getting the flu vaccine during pregnancy is not only safe, but also *highly recommended*. If you were to get the flu while pregnant, you would have a higher risk of serious illness — and even death — than getting the flu at any other time. Getting the flu vaccine won't cause a miscarriage and will keep you and your baby safe, both before and after birth.

Bottom line: You did nothing wrong. You did nothing to make this happen.

IT'S NOT YOUR FAULT

Patients come to my miscarriage clinic at all stages of the process, from freshly receiving the diagnosis to seeing me weeks after it's over. I make sure to cover the list of things that *don't* cause pregnancy loss. I always say, "It's OK to be sad, but it's *not* OK to feel guilty." Nine times out of 10, their shoulders slump with relief, and they rattle off the list of activities and behaviors that they've been secretly fearing had caused their miscarriage.

Almost all the patients I care for think that somehow the loss is their fault. They may feel like their actions led to the miscarriage — or worse, their partners or their parents or a friend implied or outright accused them of being irresponsible. The only thing worse than losing a pregnancy is thinking that it's your fault. Society is often quick to blame pregnant people for a bad outcome, and all this does is make a bad situation worse.

We can't control the outcome of a pregnancy any more than we can completely control when we get pregnant in the first place. Your pregnancy loss is not your fault.

WHAT DOES HAVING A MISCARRIAGE MEAN?

Having a miscarriage simply means that this one time of getting pregnant didn't work out.

But there's a whole list of things that it also doesn't mean:

It doesn't mean you're not healthy.

A miscarriage isn't a sign that something's wrong with you or you're sick.

It doesn't mean you can't have a healthy baby.

It's scary when a miscarriage happens, especially when it's your first pregnancy. But the odds are strong that your next pregnancy will be healthy.

It doesn't mean that you're not meant to be a parent.

Being a parent or having another child may be something that you've wanted for a long time. Some of my patients interpret a miscarriage as a sign that they're not meant to have a baby or another baby. Let me assure you that this isn't the case. The universe isn't using your miscarriage to send you a message.

It doesn't mean that you're broken.

A miscarriage may make you feel like your body isn't capable of giving you a baby. But you are not broken. This pregnancy was not healthy. That is all this loss means.

SELF-REFLECTION ABOUT MISCARRIAGE

You may feel a whole host of emotions when you find out you're losing your pregnancy. As time passes, you may want to reflect on some of the things that came to the surface around this time.

☐ Did you know how common pregnancy loss is? Do you know anyone who has had a miscarriage? If you share your experience with family and friends, you may be surprised by how many of them have been through a loss.

_____

☐ Most risk factors for miscarriage are things you can't change. When you read this chapter, do you have any of the risks of pregnancy loss that might be able to be changed?

_____

☐ When you found out you were having a miscarriage, did you start to think about your actions and experiences during the pregnancy, to see if you could find a reason for the loss? Were you surprised to see how many things are *not* associated with miscarriage?

_____

_____

_____

_____

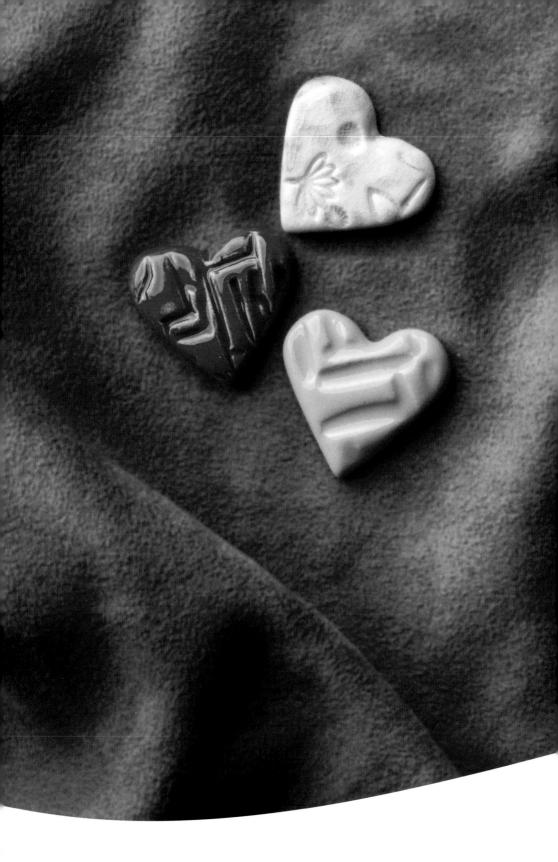

CHAPTER 2

Getting the diagnosis

Blake came to the hospital after some light vaginal spotting. She had been trying with her partner for years to have a baby, and she was so excited that this was her first. I explained to her that the pregnancy was early, her blood pregnancy hormone levels were low, and the ultrasound wasn't clear. "But am I having a miscarriage?" Blake asked anxiously. I told her we weren't sure, and we would follow her closely over the next few weeks.

The vast majority of miscarriage — 80% — happen in the first trimester. It's in these early weeks and months that there can be great uncertainty. In the first trimester, it's common to not know for sure if a miscarriage is even happening, and people are often very confused. "What do you mean you don't know? It's either fine or it's not." But there's really a big gray zone in between OK and not OK.

Miscarriages later in the pregnancy are much clearer. Sometimes a person may have bleeding. Other times, we might discover it during an ultrasound. That's the *only* good thing about a later miscarriage — there's no uncertainty. We always know it's happening.

ⓘ MEDICINE-TO-ENGLISH TRANSLATION

These basic terms will be helpful for you to understand as you read this chapter.

Cervix. The opening to your womb (uterus), at the inside end of your vagina, that needs to dilate or open to allow delivery of the baby and placenta.

Crown-rump length. Measurement from the top of the baby's head to its bum, measured from the side when the baby is curled up in the shape of a comma.

Embryo. A baby in the earliest stage of development. From shortly after fertilization of the egg by the sperm until eight weeks after conception (10 weeks of pregnancy).

Fetus. The baby inside the uterus after the first 10 weeks of pregnancy.

Gestational sac. The membrane that surrounds fluid and the growing pregnancy. Also called the pregnancy sac.

Pregnancy of unknown location. You have a positive pregnancy test, but your doctor can't see the pregnancy on an ultrasound.

Sac diameter. The measurements of the pregnancy (gestational) sac. Often the technician measures the length, width and height of the sac, then takes the average of the measurements to find the mean (average) sac diameter, which shows how far along the pregnancy is.

Trimester. Refers to a three-month time period of pregnancy. The first trimester roughly corresponds to the first three months of pregnancy, and so on.

Ultrasound. Imaging technique that uses sound waves to produce images of a pregnancy in the uterus. Can help a doctor evaluate your baby's growth and development and monitor your pregnancy. Sometimes used to evaluate possible problems or help confirm a diagnosis. May be performed on your belly (transabdominal) or with a wandlike device (transducer) placed in your vagina (transvaginal).

Viable pregnancy. A pregnancy that appears to be healthy. The embryo is visible in the uterus, and if it's large enough, it has a heartbeat.

Yolk sac. Provides nutrition and blood cells to the developing embryo before the placenta is formed and can take over. Also helps form the umbilical cord. Important in early pregnancy because it's a marker of how healthy the pregnancy is and where it's located.

Most people think of pregnancy as a binary state: You're either pregnant, or you're not. So, it's understandable to think that miscarriage works the same way. But getting a diagnosis requires sifting through sometimes conflicting signs. The embryo may be present in the pregnancy sac but may not (yet?) have a heartbeat. There may be a pregnancy sac, but no embryo inside. There may not even be a pregnancy sac at all. I want to explain why the doctors aren't always sure what's happening, and what that means for your care.

THE FIRST ULTRASOUND

Normally, you don't have an ultrasound until about 11 to 13 weeks of pregnancy. As excited as you might be to see the pregnancy, to see the heartbeat and to know that you really are truly pregnant before that time, most providers will wait.

The reason to wait is not to torture you. An ultrasound later in the first trimester gives us a lot more information about the health of the fetus. Plus, ultrasounds are expensive, and in some cases not all of them will be covered by your insurance. Your doctors wait until the results of the scan actually influence your care. Consequently, it means that you generally don't get a planned ultrasound any earlier than around three months.

At your first prenatal visit, your doctor will likely perform an internal exam with his or her fingers, with one hand on the lower part of your belly and two fingers inside your vagina. This allows the doctor to feel the actual size of your uterus. This is the first way to figure out how far along the pregnancy is. Doctors compare the size of your uterus to the first day of your last menstrual period (LMP).

Most of the time, the size of your uterus corresponds with how far the doctor thinks the pregnancy has progressed based on

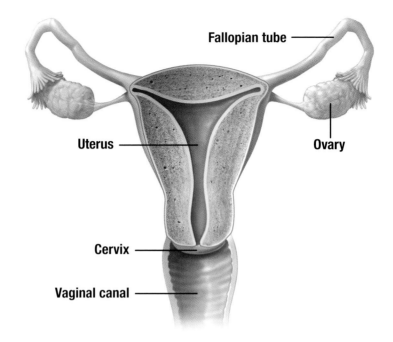

Fallopian tube

Uterus

Ovary

Cervix

Vaginal canal

Internal female anatomy. During an internal vaginal exam, your doctor can feel your cervix at the end of the vagina and can feel your uterus by placing the other hand on top of your belly.

your period. But if your uterus feels like a different size, either smaller or larger than how far along you're supposed to be, the doctor will often order an ultrasound. Sometimes, if your last menstrual period is uncertain or if you have irregular periods, you will also receive an early ultrasound.

If your uterus is bigger than the doctor expects, this often means one of two things: Either you are farther along in the pregnancy than you realized, or you have more than one fetus in there — oh my!

But if your uterus is smaller than expected, that could be a sign that the pregnancy stopped growing some time ago. This small uterus measurement may be the first sign of a miscarriage.

The other trigger for an early ultrasound is bleeding or cramping in the early months of pregnancy. While bleeding in early pregnancy is common, up to half the pregnancies with bleeding end up as a pregnancy loss of some kind. Same with cramping. While mild menstrual-type cramping is typical, sharp pain especially on one side of your pelvis instead of in the middle warrants an ultrasound.

The ultrasound experience

Some doctors perform an ultrasound themselves in their offices. Other practices will have you scanned first by an ultrasound technician, either in your regular doctor's office or in an

---

WHEN DID MY PREGNANCY BEGIN?

Doctors use a different description for how far along you are in your pregnancy from what you may be expecting. While most people think about pregnancies as lasting nine months, doctors think of pregnancies as lasting 40 weeks, which is closer to 10 months. That's because we "date" the gestational age of a pregnancy from the first day of your last period. This may seem quite odd, since no one actually gets pregnant on the first period day! Doctors use it because it's one day you know for sure, rather than guessing which day you had your egg-met-sperm moment.

What does this mean for things like trimesters? Roughly speaking, the first trimester lasts nearly 14 weeks, and the second trimester ends around 28 weeks. Ask your doctor if you need how far you are in your pregnancy described in terms you're more comfortable with.

---

ultrasound unit in a hospital. The technician or doctor will most often perform the ultrasound in two ways:

First, they'll use a probe on your belly, with jelly that looks like hair gel. This scans your uterus and the pregnancy inside.

Second, for early pregnancies, the best view of the uterus and the pregnancy comes from a transvaginal ultrasound, which is one that happens through the vagina. When you first catch a glimpse of the ultrasound probe, you might think, *No way are you putting that thing inside me,* because the probe looks ginormous. However, only about 5 inches of the probe goes inside your body. Once the ultrasound probe is inside, it's not comfortable, but it should not be painful — it feels like a speculum exam. Looking at the uterus through a transvaginal ultrasound gives the technician up close and personal pictures of your ovaries, uterus and the pregnancy itself.

When a technician performs this ultrasound, they may see one of four different things. The first scenario that they may see is a healthy pregnancy in the uterus, with what the doctors call fetal cardiac activity, and you will call a heartbeat (see "Embryonic 'heartbeat'" on page 34), as will I for simplicity's sake throughout the rest of this book. This is when the tech may print out pictures for you and say, "Congratulations!"

The second thing technicians may see is a pregnancy sac in the uterus, with the very faint beginnings of an embryo forming — but no heartbeat. This can mean one of two things: Either the pregnancy is quite early, around four or five weeks, and the embryo doesn't yet have a detectable heartbeat. Or the pregnancy may be heading toward miscarriage.

The third situation is when the technician sees a pregnancy sac but doesn't see anything inside it. An embryo may still develop — it may be simply too early to see anything — but it's possible that an embryo will never appear.

EMBRYONIC 'HEARTBEAT'

When a pregnancy is at the embryonic stage at less than eight weeks of development, we may see a pulsation in the embryo that the health care team will tell you is a "heartbeat." But what you think of as a heart doesn't develop until much further along in the pregnancy. At this stage, there is a small clump of cells showing electrical activity, which causes the firefly-like flicker on the ultrasound screen. It's a positive sign for development of the pregnancy, but it isn't technically a heartbeat yet. Though for someone anxious about the possibility of miscarriage, this electrical spark may make your own heart leap with joy.

The last situation is the most frustrating: The technician isn't sure if there's a sac inside the uterus. This can mean that the pregnancy is superearly — what I like to call being "20 minutes" pregnant — or it could mean that a miscarriage is going to happen. At this stage, if you have a positive pregnancy test but your doctor can't see the pregnancy on ultrasound, you have a mysterious-sounding pregnancy of unknown location.

What the ultrasound means

Ultrasound technicians likely won't explain what they're seeing. (Technicians would make excellent poker players.) They're going to give the details about the ultrasound to the doctor, who reviews the images before saying anything to you. The doctor may repeat the test if there's uncertainty about what the pictures are showing. Hopefully, you'll be able to get information while you're at the hospital or office, but the doctor may call you later with the results. This delay can mean an uncomfortable wait.

What the heck is a "chemical pregnancy"?

This is not a test-tube baby, or one conceived after a few drinks (or hits). A chemical pregnancy is one that has not progressed far enough to create tissue visible on an ultrasound. In these pregnancies, the egg and sperm joined, and the resulting embryo implanted and started making pregnancy hormones, but the pregnancy rapidly stopped developing.

Because they sound a little similar, sometimes there's confusion between a *chemical pregnancy* and a *clinical miscarriage*, which is a pregnancy that *can* be documented by ultrasound. Confusing matters further, sometimes these are referred to as *chemical losses* and *clinical losses*, respectively. I know — unfortunate naming, for sure.

Why does this matter? These two different kinds of losses are treated very differently when you experience more than one of them. Two or more clinical pregnancy losses — referred to as recurrent pregnancy losses — are a *miscarriage* problem, while many doctors consider multiple chemical pregnancy losses an *infertility* problem. Chapter 9 offers more detail about recurrent loss.

From a doctor's standpoint, three things could be happening:

1. You can have a pregnancy inside your uterus — what doctors call a viable pregnancy.
2. You may have an unusual type of miscarriage called an ectopic pregnancy, where the pregnancy is growing outside the uterus rather than inside it (see Chapter 10).

3. Your pregnancy is inside your uterus, but the technician suspects — or knows — you're having a miscarriage.

By seeing a pregnancy sac or an embryo inside your uterus, your doctor can tell you how far along your pregnancy is. This is called "dating" your pregnancy. Once your doctor knows when the pregnancy started, he or she knows exactly what things should look like at different stages at follow-up exams and ultrasounds. So with future ultrasounds, we can tell if the pregnancy is growing normally, or if there is arrested development at some point and the pregnancy turns into a miscarriage.

An ultrasound can give your doctor a lot of information and answer what triggered the ultrasound exam in the first place:

- **If your uterus felt too small or too large,** the ultrasound determines how far along the pregnancy is, including your due date.
- **If you have bleeding or pain,** an ultrasound ideally shows if there's a healthy pregnancy in the uterus. If so, your doctor will follow up with another ultrasound in a few weeks to make sure that the pregnancy grows appropriately. Your doctor will likely tell you not to worry, which I know is hard to do. Then the waiting begins.

If your ultrasound can't pinpoint **where the pregnancy is,** the doctor's next mission is to make sure that the pregnancy is in the uterus and not somewhere else, like in your fallopian tube (see Chapter 10). You'll likely get a blood test to measure the level of pregnancy hormones in your blood. You'll have this test at least twice, approximately 48 hours apart, and repeated as needed, along with more ultrasounds as indicated.

Progression of a pregnancy onscreen

Technicians and the doctors look for four things in your ultrasound (see the first three on the next page).

PROGRESSION OF AN EARLY PREGNANCY ON ULTRASOUND

Early in pregnancy, you will first see A) the pregnancy (gestational) sac appear, followed by B) the yolk sac, and finally C) the embryo.

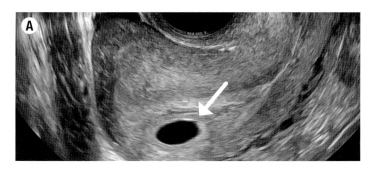

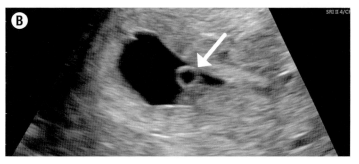

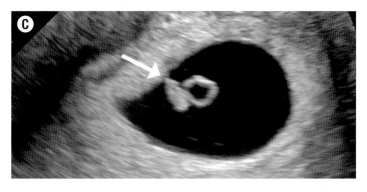

- The first thing to appear is the pregnancy (or gestational) sac in your uterus. This looks like a black circle in the middle of a gray blob.
- Second, they're waiting to see a yolk sac. This looks like a white ring in the middle of this black circle.
- Next, they're looking for what we call the fetal pole. This is the actual embryo developing. It may be shaped like a medication capsule. It will take the shape of a peanut as it grows.
- Finally, they are waiting for the embryo to have a heartbeat.

These pregnancy signs usually appear in this order over the course of about two to three weeks. Sometimes you can see a heartbeat before you see an embryo, which is pretty amazing.

When doctors say they're not sure what's happening, it's common to wonder, *What do you mean you're not sure? What do you mean you can't tell me what's happening?*

With a single ultrasound, your doctor has only a snapshot in time of what's happening in your uterus. Sometimes we can only diagnose a miscarriage by following you over the course of days or weeks to see the changes happening inside your body. Especially when we see someone before five weeks of pregnancy, and all these visual signs are not yet present, we have to wait to see if they all develop as they should.

WHAT YOUR DOCTOR IS WAITING FOR

The best sign that we hope to see on an ultrasound is an embryo with a heartbeat. Once we see a heartbeat in a pregnancy, your chances of miscarriage drop to between 1% and 11%. The chances never reach zero, of course, but until we see an embryo with a heartbeat, there is much more uncertainty.

Sometimes you'll see an embryo with a heartbeat on one ultrasound, and then on another, the heartbeat is gone. That is a definite sign you're having a miscarriage. It's natural to want to get another ultrasound when this happens, just to make sure. But once the heartbeat has disappeared, we never see it come back.

Sometimes the pregnancy sac will grow, but an embryo never appears. Or an embryo appears and is tiny — less than 5 millimeters — and never develops a heartbeat at all. The way doctors then know for sure is by doing multiple ultrasounds, usually 7 to 14 days apart, depending on what your first ultrasound showed. They're looking for signs of "interval change" — giving the pregnancy a chance to grow. If there's no change on the next ultrasound, meaning an embryo or heartbeat hasn't appeared, you're having a miscarriage.

During this period of uncertainty, it's understandable to want an ultrasound every day to see what's happening and to get more information. The best thing you can do is to try to be patient and follow your doctor's schedule of tests. Your doctor isn't making you wait because he or she is busy, I promise. Your doctor wants to make sure

My next ultrasound isn't for 10 days—I don't want to wait that long!

that every time you have a test, whether it's a blood test or an ultrasound, it's providing usable information. Ultrasounds performed too closely together in time don't help us reach a diagnosis — it's only by waiting a week or more that we can interpret what we're seeing on the screen.

Make sure that your doctor explains to you clearly why certain tests are ordered, what they mean, and how you can contact the office to get the results of the tests as soon as they come back from the lab. Because you're getting so much information at these visits, you may want to bring a support person with you. You could bring your partner, your friend or your mom — anyone who can help you "get" what the doctor is saying. I sometimes see a support person for my patient taking notes

ULTRASOUND DIAGNOSIS OF MISCARRIAGE

Doctors have highly specific criteria for diagnosing a miscarriage by ultrasound. If you're really into numbers and you've been closely following the details of your ultrasound exams, here are several signs that strongly indicate you're having a miscarriage (though these signs aren't definitive):

- An empty gestational sac with no visible embryo
- A mean sac diameter (average length of the sac) of 16 to 24 mm and no embryo
- Absence of an embryo 6 weeks or more after your last menstrual period
- Absence of embryo with heartbeat 7 to 13 days after a scan that showed a gestational sac *without* a yolk sac
- Absence of embryo with heartbeat 7 to 10 days after a scan that showed a gestational sac *with* a yolk sac
- An enlarged yolk sac that's more than 7 mm in diameter
- A gestational sac that's small in relation to the size of the embryo (less than 5 mm difference between mean sac diameter and crown–rump length)
- An embryo that's less than 7 mm and has no heartbeat

These ultrasound findings indicate for sure that the pregnancy is lost:

- A mean sac diameter of 25 mm or larger and no embryo
- Absence of embryo with heartbeat two weeks or more after a scan that showed a gestational sac *without* a yolk sac
- Absence of embryo with heartbeat 11 days or more after a scan that showed a gestational sac *with* a yolk sac
- A crown-rump length of the embryo of 7 mm or larger, with no heartbeat

during the visit, and even asking questions of their own. This gives me confidence that my patient is going to have a greater understanding of what we talked about and is less likely to miss something important. I actually do this myself — even doctors, when they're patients, can forget to ask the questions they have or will not end up hearing everything their doctors say during a visit. Thank goodness for getting written end-of-visit instructions!

This uncertainty around the future can be extremely frustrating, when all you want is to be sure of what's happening. But you will be as sure as your doctor is. Your doctor will never keep information from you about what's happening in the pregnancy. As soon as the doctor knows, you'll know, too.

WHILE YOU'RE WAITING

During this time, it's important to take care of yourself physically and emotionally. Physically, there's nothing you can't do. You should still have your daily cup of coffee, and you should still go for your morning run. You can even have sex. None of these things are going to change what's going to happen with your pregnancy. As I discussed in the last chapter, there's nothing that you can do to make the pregnancy healthier, or to save it if it's not healthy. The best thing you can do is to keep up your regular routines.

Since this is a really hard time, you also want to take care of yourself emotionally. Have someone else clean your house, get takeout for dinner, and skip the holiday cards this year. Give yourself permission to slow down and feel your feelings.

If you want to, confide in people who support you. Letting people know what's going on can get you the help you need. I would tell them exactly

What do I tell my family?

what you know (and what your doctor knows) — that you're pregnant, but you aren't sure if the pregnancy is healthy or if it's going to develop, and you need more testing to be sure.

Don't get anybody involved who is going to bombard you with questions, blame you or make you feel guilty, catastrophize, or give you advice about preventing a miscarriage. This will not help you. This uncertainty is why I caution my patients to not tell their *entire* world too quickly when a pregnancy test is positive. Telling vague acquaintances that you could be having a miscarriage is only likely to invite insensitive and uninformed suggestions.

On the other hand, sharing your miscarriage experience more widely could go a long way to help reverse the stigma around discussing loss. Think of the bravery Chrissy Teigen showed

MISCARRIAGE IN THE EMERGENCY ROOM

About half a million people in the U.S. are seen in an emergency room (ER) because of vaginal bleeding in pregnancy, and nearly 200,000 people receive a diagnosis of early pregnancy loss each year there. Countless others are diagnosed with an ectopic pregnancy in an ER.

Emergency rooms are busy places, filled with people who need urgent medical help. If you've ever been in an emergency room, you've probably witnessed the high amount of stress everyone is feeling — providers included. In this fast-paced environment, emergency room technicians are focused on treating and stabilizing people in often-dire situations, moving from one person to the next to treat people as quickly and efficiently as possible, with as much care and concern as they can offer, in the time that they have available.

If you're diagnosed with a pregnancy loss in an emergency room and you feel as if you're rushed through the process, know that it's not because your situation doesn't matter. Emergency room technicians are doing the best that they can to care for people in a variety of devastating circumstances. And while this medical care is top-notch, sometimes the emotional care can be less than we want it to be.

If you need to call your doctor because of concerns about your pregnancy, and he or she suggests going to the emergency room, ask if there's another option. You may be able to be seen in your doctor's office, if an ultrasound machine is available. Or your doctor may be able to send you to a women's health triage unit, perhaps on a hospital's labor and delivery unit, where you can see providers who are experienced with early pregnancy symptoms.

when she shared her pregnancy loss on Instagram and Twitter. We need more conversations about miscarriage for people to understand how common this is. But you should not bear the weight of responsibility for society's awakening to miscarriage on your shoulders. Only tell who you want to.

WHAT YOU MAY HEAR

There are many terms you may hear a doctor use when you're told that you're having a first trimester miscarriage. Here's what each one means.

- **Anembryonic gestation.** There is a pregnancy in your uterus, but there is no embryo. Sometimes called a blighted ovum.
- **Embryonic or fetal demise.** There is an embryo or fetus in the gestational sac, but there is no heartbeat when there should be one.
- **Incomplete abortion.** Your cervix is dilated, and some but not all the pregnancy tissue has already passed out of your uterus.
- **Inevitable abortion.** Your cervix is dilated, and the pregnancy tissue will pass out of your uterus soon.
- **Missed abortion.** The pregnancy has stopped developing, possibly a few weeks ago. Your uterus hasn't begun to expel the pregnancy tissue yet, and you've likely had little to no bleeding or cramping.
- **Spontaneous abortion.** Officially, you've had a miscarriage, where your body passed all the pregnancy tissue without medication or a procedure. Some doctors will call a fetal demise a spontaneous abortion, even if you haven't started bleeding yet. Unofficially, doctors may refer to any miscarriage as a spontaneous abortion, including one that needs medication or a procedure to complete it.

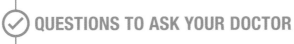 QUESTIONS TO ASK YOUR DOCTOR

Bring this list of questions with you to your first doctor's appointment. Take notes and check off the questions as you go.

☐ What can you see on the ultrasound? What do you expect to see, based on how far along I am?

_____

☐ What's the best way to follow up: with blood tests, ultrasounds or both?

_____

☐ When do I need to get the next test?

_____

☐ What are you hoping to see with this next test? What are the other possibilities of what you might see?

_____

☐ If I need to get multiple blood tests, do I need to come back to your office or the hospital? Or can I go to a lab that is closer to my home or job?

_____

☐ Do you have any concerns that the pregnancy may not be in the uterus?

_____

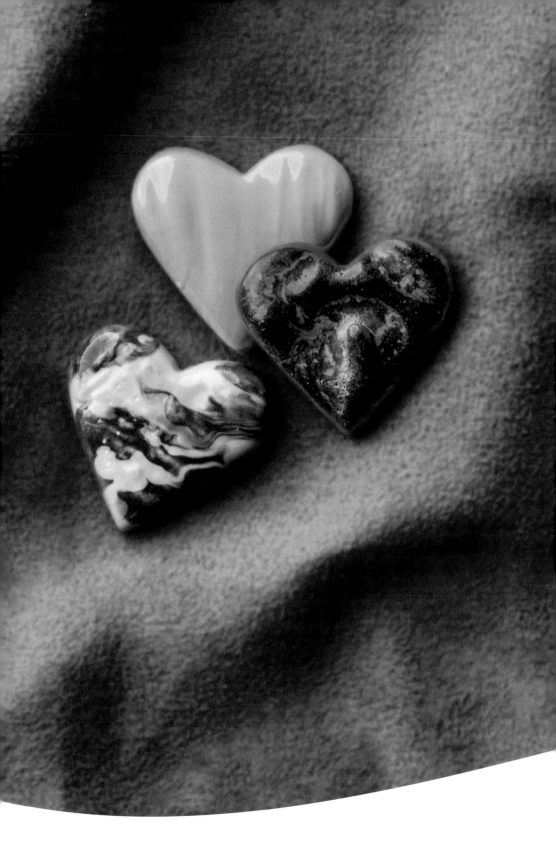

CHAPTER 3

Choosing your path for first trimester loss

Camilla, a young woman pregnant for the first time, had an uneventful pregnancy until her routine first trimester ultrasound showed a fetal demise at eight weeks. Three days later, she saw me so that we could review her options for management. Camilla wasn't ready to make a decision that day and wanted to review what I told her with her boyfriend and her mother. She told me, "I want to be in control as much as possible over what happens next."

Once your doctor confirms the diagnosis of a miscarriage, you'll often have time to think before you have to decide what to do next. Let me clarify that I'm talking about *first trimester* pregnancy loss in these next few chapters. I will address the more complicated scenarios of second and third trimester losses in their own chapters. I'm also talking primarily about *missed abortions,* in which the pregnancy has stopped developing but the process of the miscarriage hasn't yet begun.

In brief, you have three options with a first trimester miscarriage: You can wait until the miscarriage happens naturally, use medication or have a surgical procedure. Another way to think about it is choosing between *passive* management — a fancy term for doing nothing (watching and waiting) — and *active* management, where you take steps to do something to help the miscarriage complete.

Before considering the options available to you, take time to care for yourself. After the diagnosis and as the miscarriage is happening, take these steps:

- Take notes during your visit with your doctor. It's easy to forget things in your shock and grief.
- Write down questions to ask your doctor as they come up.
- If you can, bring your partner or a friend to your appointments for emotional support (and a second set of ears).
- Figure out the best timing of completion of the miscarriage for you.
- Share what is happening with your support network.

- If you have children at home, organize child care during your miscarriage treatment.
- Plan treatment around your job as much as possible, taking sick days or paid leave, if you can.
- Stock up on what gives you comfort: favorite foods, trashy magazines, movies, library books, podcasts, music.
- Make no commitments to anyone outside of your closest friends and family members.

OPTION 1: EXPECTANT MANAGEMENT

The first option is to do nothing. Doctors call this expectant management. With this option, you let your body handle the miscarriage at its own pace. Most times with a first trimester miscarriage, your body eventually passes the pregnancy on its own. This approach is a good choice for people who prefer as natural an experience with their miscarriage as possible.

The benefits of waiting it out are straightforward: You avoid medical intervention and let the pregnancy end on its own. Once the pregnancy has stopped growing and the signals to continue the pregnancy are no longer there, your uterus will expel the pregnancy tissue. You may have fewer doctor's visits and fewer ultrasounds and blood draws with this option.

The risks of expectant management are just like the risks of active management. Bleeding that becomes heavy enough to require urgent medical attention is always a risk. The pregnancy also might not pass on its own and require additional medical intervention. This happens more often with a miscarriage over 10 weeks' gestation, so health care providers may caution you about waiting it out if your pregnancy has advanced beyond that point. The biggest risk may be that the miscarriage begins at the worst possible time — while you're at work, in church or in some other place that makes it difficult for you to take care of yourself in the way that you would want.

Patients often ask me, "How long will I have to wait?" That question can be hard to answer. When your health care provider examines you around the time of your miscarriage diagnosis, your body may show signs that a miscarriage is imminent. For instance, your cervix may be soft or partially open, or a small amount of tissue may be starting to pass. Sometimes the ultrasound can give you clues, too. The scan may show that the pregnancy sac is already starting to work its way into the cervix, which shows that your body has started the miscarriage process even if you haven't started to bleed or cramp yet.

In general, it's difficult to predict how long it may take for a miscarriage to start or finish. It may take up to eight weeks from the time of diagnosis for the miscarriage to begin, and it may take another two weeks to complete after that. That may be too long for some people to want to wait, but it's nice to know that you have the option.

OPTION 2: SURGICAL MANAGEMENT

If you're anxious to be done with the miscarriage as soon as possible, the most straightforward option is a procedure called a dilation and curettage (D&C). This kind of surgery for a first trimester miscarriage may take place in an operating room, surgical center or even a doctor's office. You may be awake or asleep. It usually takes under 10 minutes, and you will be able to go home the same day.

Here's what happens: The doctor opens your cervix with instruments called dilators. There's no cutting involved, just stretching the natural opening of your body. Then the doctor uses suction, either with a hand-operated suction device called a manual vacuum aspirator (MVA) or an electric vacuum, to remove the pregnancy. You go home the same day, and the bleeding and cramping after the procedure feels like a period. See what an MVA looks like on page 96.

With a surgical procedure, you know when and where the pregnancy is going to end. There's also a pattern for bleeding and cramping that most people experience, unlike the unpredictability of how you feel with either expectant or medical management. Surgery is also the most reliable option if it's important to collect the pregnancy tissue for chromosomal testing. And it's the only option in which you may be able to be asleep while the miscarriage is happening.

There are several risks of a D&C for a miscarriage, but each of them are quite low. They include:

- **Excessive bleeding,** which the doctor can control with medication or a minor procedure called an embolization
- **Infection,** which is treated with antibiotics
- **Perforation,** an injury to the uterus or cervix during the procedure that may require surgery to repair it
- **Retained tissue,** in which all the fetal tissue isn't removed by the procedure and you need treatment to remove it
- **Anesthesia risks,** which apply only if the procedure is performed under sedation

It's important to know that surgical procedures to complete a miscarriage are very safe. Many people worry about risking future pregnancies by not being patient for this current miscarriage to begin. Let me reassure you — a complication-free D&C procedure doesn't affect your ability to get pregnant again. Complications are most often minor, if they happen at all, and ones that impact fertility are exceedingly low.

OPTION 3: MEDICAL MANAGEMENT

You may fall somewhere in between these two options. You may not be comfortable waiting for nature to take its course but may be hesitant to undergo a surgical procedure if you don't absolutely need one. If this is how you feel, there is a third way: medical management.

With medical management, your health care provider gives you medication that you can take when you feel ready to accelerate the first trimester miscarriage process. The most effective medication, mifepristone (Mifeprex), is swallowed in the doctor's office. It starts your uterus contracting and readies it for the next medication, misoprostol (Cytotec). Misoprostol causes the lining of the uterus to slough off along with the miscarriage tissue. If your doctor doesn't have mifepristone, you'll be given misoprostol by itself. You'll place four tablets in your cheek or in your vagina the next day. Most of the time, patients begin bleeding and cramping within four hours of taking the medication. Bleeding may be heavy for several hours; then it tapers off, like a regular period. This method is best for people who want to start the miscarriage but avoid a procedure.

The risk with medical management is that while the misoprostol tablets usually begin working within four hours, sometimes they don't. It may take many hours or even days before you begin bleeding and passing the pregnancy tissue. And some people never bleed at all after a single dose of the medication. Your doctor may schedule an ultrasound several days or a week after you take the medication to make sure that the pregnancy has passed. Sometimes, a second dose of medication is required to complete the process. Overall, it can take up to a week for you to finish passing all the pregnancy tissue. This unpredictability may be a drawback.

Another drawback of medical management is that not all doctors can give mifepristone. You'll learn why in Chapter 5. Your doctor can give you just the misoprostol tablets to use, but misoprostol doesn't work quite as well when used by itself.

HOW TO CHOOSE

If you didn't know that you had options for managing a first trimester miscarriage, this list can seem overwhelming. But the options for treatment are all equally safe, and none will negatively affect your chances of getting pregnant in the future. What is different is the experience of the miscarriage.

Here are some of the factors that drive my patients' decision-making. This list can help guide you into choosing the option that's right for you.

Timing

Some people can't stand the idea of waiting and want a process they can manage as quickly as possible. Or they may have an important life event coming up — a wedding or a vacation — and don't want their miscarriage to affect their enjoyment of this event (as much as possible). For these folks, scheduling a surgical procedure is the best way to maintain control over the timing of the miscarriage. My second miscarriage, at five weeks, came on suddenly, at the start of a 24-hour shift at the hospital. I wish I'd had more control of the timing — at work was the last place I wanted to be when losing my pregnancy.

Taking action

Some of my patients want to hold on to hope, however unrealistic, that the pregnancy will be OK and that my diagnosis was wrong. They want to listen to their bodies, and will only feel OK about the loss when they start bleeding on their own. Other patients want to avoid all medical intervention and let their miscarriage happen naturally, even if the process takes longer.

Avoiding pain

Some people are anxious or even terrified about how much pain they'll be in when the miscarriage occurs. For anyone who wants to reduce pain with the miscarriage as much as possible, I recommend a surgical procedure with moderate or deep sedation. You won't have to be awake during the procedure itself, and the physical pain you'll feel when you wake up is very much like the pain you may experience with periods.

Exercising

If you're an active person, exercising may be vitally important for both your physical and mental health. You likely won't feel like heavy exercise the day of the miscarriage — no matter which method of management you choose —

Exercise is important to me. Is one approach better than another?

but the post-miscarriage recovery course is similar in terms of what you can do. I counsel my patients to continue whatever exercise regimen they were on before the loss. Just listen to your body — if you're not in pain or noticing that the bleeding has become heavy again, exercise as much as you want.

Finances

Medical bills may be the furthest thing from your mind when you're deciding how to manage your miscarriage. But the cost of medical care, even for pregnancy loss, can't easily be ignored. Medical bills depend on your insurance coverage and may come in several forms, including:
- A copay for an office visit (often $100 or less)
- The cost of medications (which may or may not be covered)
- A deductible for a surgical procedure

Just the cost of the procedure can vary wildly, depending on:
- The location of the procedure (office, surgical center or operating room)

- How much and what type of anesthesia you receive
- Whether all the health care providers are in network for your insurance (including the anesthesiologist)
- Any medical conditions you may have that affect your care

If you're fortunate to have good health insurance, it should cover most of the costs of your treatment. If you have insurance at all, it should cover at least some of the costs of your treatment. But if you're uninsured, you may want to reduce your medical costs as much as possible, and expectant management may be the financially smartest way to go.

Another cost to consider is the genetic testing of the pregnancy tissue. Tissue analysis may not be covered by your insurance until you're having your third miscarriage. The costs vary depending on where you live, but this testing can cost hundreds or even thousands of dollars, so ask your doctor or your insurance company before this test is ordered.

Ask your doctor's office to help you figure out what the charges would be for the treatment options you're considering. You don't want to be facing surprise medical bills at the time you're supposed to be healing from your loss. It's possible that your doctor's office will refer you to your insurance company for this information. If this is the case, ask someone at your doctor's office for the diagnosis codes used for your care. You'll have a much better experience on the phone with an agent if you're both speaking the same (insurance) language.

Testing

Your doctor may recommend performing a chromosomal analysis of the pregnancy tissue to try to detect an abnormality that explains the miscarriage. If this is important to you, the best option is a surgical procedure. This way, the doctor can send the tissue directly to the lab for analysis. But if you have your heart set on *not* having a procedure, the doctor can give you a specimen cup to collect pregnancy tissue or large blood clots. It's not as reliable as collecting tissue during surgery, but this method has worked for some of my patients. Find details on how to collect the tissue in Chapter 4.

If your doctor doesn't bring up genetic testing, you may be unsure if you should ask about it. You may want to consider genetic testing of the pregnancy tissue if:
• You've had more than one miscarriage
• There was a fetal abnormality seen on the ultrasound
• You have a family history of miscarriage or of chromosomal abnormalities
• You want to learn all you can about the loss

Testing is generally done on tissue or fluid taken before, during or after a miscarriage. This testing helps show if the pregnancy had the correct number and configuration of chromosomes. If an abnormality is detected, it can explain why the miscarriage occurred.

You may have to wait up to 6 to 8 weeks to get results, and your doctor or your genetic counselor will be able to explain what the findings mean.

You may *not* want testing if:
• It's your first loss, and a chromosomal abnormality wouldn't change any of your plans about getting pregnant again
• It's not covered by your insurance
• It means more to you to have expectant management or medical management, which reduces the chance of successful testing (because you may not be able to identify the pregnancy tissue to send for the testing)

It's also possible that you'll wait weeks for the results, just to find that the testing can't give you an answer. Talk with your doctor about what's recommended for your particular loss.

Safety

Even after I present the choices as all being low-risk, patients will often ask me, "What's the safest choice?" Luckily, having a miscarriage doesn't entail serious risks for the vast majority of people, no matter which method of management you choose. It's not any riskier to your health to choose a procedure over waiting it out, for instance.

That said, there's no way to guarantee there won't be a complication with *any* path you choose. Each method of miscarriage treatment has its own set of risks, but these risks are very, very low. I remind my patients that *everything* in life involves risks,

---

TESTING PERFORMED BEFORE ALMOST ALL MISCARRIAGES

Regardless of what treatment method you choose, your doctor will likely ask you to have blood drawn for testing. This is done to show:
- If you're anemic or at risk of needing a blood transfusion after the miscarriage.
- Your blood type — in particular, if your blood type is Rh-positive or Rh-negative. If it's the latter, you'll need an injection of Rhogam, a special medication to prevent complications in future pregnancies. Rhogam is given as soon as you have bleeding in a pregnancy, on the day of a surgical procedure or within 72 hours of beginning medical management of a miscarriage.

If you had these labs drawn with a slew of other prenatal labs at your first visit of the pregnancy, you may not need them drawn again.

---

from using a tampon (toxic shock syndrome!) to driving a car (accidents!) to having sex (sexually transmitted infections!). Overall, for most people, each management option is as safe as the others. Choose the path that feels best for you.

When I have this conversation with my patients, many tell me that they have read some scary things online about miscarriage. It's understandable that the first place many people turn to for information is the internet. But please remember that what you read online or hear from your friends and family may not apply to your own situation — or be accurate at all. Your search engine is not board-certified and is completely unaccountable, so verify any information with your doctor.

CHANGING YOUR TREATMENT — OR YOUR MIND

It's common to use multiple methods of treatment during the same first trimester miscarriage. That's because things don't always proceed as planned. I had a patient who wanted a natural miscarriage but didn't want to wait up to six weeks. She waited it out for two weeks and followed up with me. Since she hadn't yet started bleeding, she took mifepristone in my office, carried the misoprostol tablets home with her and took them on Saturday to have her miscarriage on the weekend.

Another patient started with medical management to begin her miscarriage. When I saw her at her follow-up visit, the ultrasound showed that she still had pregnancy tissue in her uterus. Frustrated that the misoprostol didn't work completely, she elected surgery to finish the process. Another patient in the same situation decided to wait to see if the remaining tissue would pass on its own over the next few days, and it did.

I've also had many patients who plan to have surgery, but before the day of the procedure, they start bleeding and pass the pregnancy on their own. Know that you can choose which way to start the process, but you might adjust your plan based on how you're feeling and how your body acts.

WHEN YOU'RE NOT GIVEN A CHOICE

Your doctor will consider many factors about your individual situation before offering you choices for what to do next. After reading about these options, you may be surprised if your doctor only presents you with one option for management. I try to give my patients the choice of all three options for a first trimester miscarriage, but sometimes will make recommendations based on their situations.

For example, I encourage patients who are beyond 10 weeks to choose a surgical procedure because I believe it has fewer risks of excessive bleeding compared with the other two choices. If a patient has waited out the miscarriage for over two months, I'll suggest a procedure for the same reason. And if a patient's cervix is dilated (open), I may suggest either watchful waiting or using medication, as I think the miscarriage will likely be over soon. But in the end, I believe that all people should choose their own path. They are the ones who have to experience the miscarriage in that particular way.

There's no one right answer for all people every time. Some of my patients who've had multiple miscarriages have made different choices depending on what was happening with their lives and bodies at the time. Ask all the questions you have before making your decision.

If your doctor gives you only one choice for your miscarriage and it's not the path that you prefer, speak up. Ask if another way to manage the loss is possible, or why those other options aren't good choices for you right now. It may be that your doctor isn't comfortable with one or more of these options. If this is the situation, ask if one of his or her partners can care for you

COMPARING THE OPTIONS

Option	Expectant management	
Where does it happen?	On your own at home	
How long does it take?	Can take up to 8 weeks	
Will I need follow-up care?	May need only one follow-up visit, or more if the pregnancy doesn't pass on its own	
How long will bleeding last?	Bleeding for up to 6 weeks on and off	
What are the risks?	Unexpected bleeding, heavy bleeding that needs emergent treatment, or it doesn't work	
Will I need additional care?	About 1 in 5 people needs a surgical procedure	

	Medical management	Surgical management
	On your own at home	In the office or operating room
	Can take from one day to a week	Takes no more than a day
	May need one or more follow-up visits, depending on the success of the medication	Follow-up is not often needed
	Bleeding for up to 3 weeks on and off	Bleeding for up to 2 weeks on and off
	Heavy bleeding that needs emergent treatment, or it doesn't work	Heavy bleeding that needs emergent treatment, infection, injury to the cervix or uterus, retained tissue that needs a second procedure to remove
	5%-20% chance of needing a surgical procedure	Less than 1% chance of needing a second surgical procedure

in the way you prefer, or if you can be referred to another doctor. If it's safe, you should have your choice.

You may be told you're having a miscarriage during an ultrasound when the doctor comes in to tell you the news. You may be waiting for a phone call at home to confirm what you already know. Either way, take time to process the diagnosis and reflect on what you want to do next. You don't have to make a quick decision — take the time you need.

PREPARING FOR THE MISCARRIAGE TO BEGIN

Whichever way you manage your miscarriage, there are steps you can take to make the process more comfortable:
- Buy menstrual pads and liners, if you're usually a tampon or cup user, or have someone buy them for you.
- Buy an over-the-counter nonsteroidal anti-inflammatory drug like ibuprofen (Advil, Motrin IB, others) or naproxen sodium (Aleve) if your doctor hasn't given you a prescription for pain medication. You shouldn't need opioid medication like codeine or oxycodone (OxyContin, Roxicodone, others). But if your pain can't be controlled with these medications, call your doctor.
- Have a medical pad, an old towel, or a bed liner of some sort on hand to protect your mattress.
- Use a heating pad or hot water bottle on your lower belly or back (wherever you're feeling pain) or take a hot bath or shower. You can also make a homemade heat pack by putting dry rice into a clean sock, knotting the end and microwaving it for 30 seconds. Reheat as often as needed.
- Sleep as much as you can. Coping is much harder when you're tired.

Though we can't control *when* a pregnancy ends, in most cases, you should have some control over *how* it ends. The next three chapters offer information to help you make your decision.

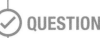 **QUESTIONS TO ASK YOUR DOCTOR**

Bring this list of questions to your appointment to ask regarding your treatment options. Take notes and check off the questions as you go.

☐ When do you think the miscarriage happened?

_____

☐ How long do you think it would take my body to complete the miscarriage if I don't do anything to help it along?

_____

☐ If I want to wait out the miscarriage, how can I follow up with the office with questions? How soon should I come back to the office for a visit?

_____

☐ If I want a procedure, will you be the one to perform it? How soon can we schedule it? Where will the procedure happen — in the office, in the hospital or somewhere else? What are my options for anesthesia?

_____

☐ If I want to use medical management, what medications do you prescribe?

_____

PART 2

Experiencing

Now that we've traveled through the confusing and shocking part of a first trimester miscarriage diagnosis, let's walk through the first trimester miscarriage experience.

These chapters outline all the experiences of a first trimester loss. You'll learn how to prepare for it, what it feels like when it's happening, and what to expect when it's over.

CHAPTER 4

Expectant management: Waiting it out

Destiny called me an hour before her appointment. "I don't know if I need to come in this morning," she told me. "I think I've passed the pregnancy, but I don't know for sure." She reported having heavy cramps and a lot of bleeding. "I saw a lot of blood clots come out, so I searched for 'miscarriage blood clots' online. A woman posted pictures of her miscarriage, and her blood clots look like mine did. Does that mean the miscarriage is over?"

You've made the decision to let your first trimester miscarriage happen on its own, known as expectant management, in which you wait for the miscarriage to happen naturally. If your body is ready, the process could start soon — but it could also take time. Let's talk about what it feels like along the way.

MISCARRIAGE, STEP BY STEP

The longest part of the miscarriage is waiting for it to start, which may take up to eight weeks. While you're waiting, you may not feel different in any way. Some people find that their pregnancy symptoms end during this time — they're no longer nauseous, their breasts aren't tender, and they get some energy back. But these symptoms may stick around until the miscarriage is over. You may also start to have mild cramping or spotting in the days leading up to the start of the process.

For some people, the miscarriage begins gradually. Mild cramping slowly intensifies, and spotting becomes light bleeding and then heavier bleeding. But sometimes, the miscarriage comes on suddenly — one minute you're feeling fine, the next you're overtaken by serious pain or heavy bleeding, or both.

I recommend to my patients that if you're waiting it out, you need to be prepared with an exit strategy. You may not want to travel to remote places without a bathroom, for instance, or to be on an outing or trip with people who don't know what's happening. You might need to go to work or school and participate in the typical activities of life while you're waiting, since you don't know when the bleeding might start.

But you should have a plan if your miscarriage starts in earnest. For example, you may want to leave work when the pain or bleeding worsens, and that might mean giving your boss a heads-up or getting someone to cover your work for you. And you absolutely want to have maxi pads close at hand during this time.

Just like the rest of pregnancy, each person experiences miscarriages differently. Some people have physical symptoms similar to their periods. Others have much more intense cramping that makes them want to stay in bed. Bleeding also can be worse than your usual period, with the passing of clots and a brisk flow. The worst of the bleeding and cramping most often lasts 2 to 8 hours, then tapers off into bleeding like a period. It's during this time of heavy bleeding that the pregnancy passes.

You may be wondering: *What will I see if I pass the pregnancy at home? Will I see the baby?* It's rare for even doctors to see any part of the baby before 10 weeks' gestation, so if you're having a miscarriage at home before that point, it's exceedingly unlikely you would see anything recognizable among the blood clots and small amounts of tan-gray tissue.

If you are losing your pregnancy at 10 weeks' gestation or later, it's possible that you'll see the baby pass. Some patients have told me about seeing the baby and, because they were prepared for this to happen, said it wasn't shocking and didn't make them sad. But if you think that seeing the baby would be distressing, talk with your doctor about your options.

Since the miscarriage process may have been preceded by lighter bleeding and cramping, you may feel like you've been bleeding for weeks. It's typical for this process to take time, lasting as long as three weeks.

That might not seem helpful, since there are many ways you might feel. But in the end, everything you're feeling is normal.

Managing pain

If your doctor doesn't prescribe pain medication, the best way to take over-the-counter medications (assuming you're not allergic or can't take them for another reason) is to start before the pain becomes severe. Take your first dose as soon as you feel cramping begin. You may even want to take your first dose as soon as you see spotting. The sooner you take medication, the more effective it is.

A MISCARRIAGE KIT

Some people may want to not only know exactly when the pregnancy passes but also see the tissue itself. I tell these patients to gather the following before their bleeding begins:
- A bedpan or a "hat" that sits on the toilet under the seat. This is usually used to collect and measure urine. Your doctor may be able to give you one from the office, or you can buy one from a medical supply store or online.
- A mesh strainer, the kind you usually find at a dollar store that gets the pulp out of orange juice.
- Disposable medical or dishwashing gloves.
- A jar with a lid or a specimen cup from your doctor.
- A bottle of saline or contact lens solution, if you're not comfortable rinsing the tissue in your sink.

Once bleeding becomes heavier than spotting — more like a period, or they start passing clots — I recommend that they use the bedpan or hat whenever they use the toilet. The aim is to capture as much of the blood as possible. The blood and clots can then be poured into the strainer over a sink. As you rinse the strainer with water or saline, you can tap or massage the clots to break them up and see if there is tissue inside.

For pain management, you have three options, all of which are available at your local drugstore or grocery store:

- **Ibuprofen** (Advil, Motrin IB, others). Take 600 mg (three 200-mg tablets or capsules) every six hours, **or** 800 mg (four 200-mg tablets or capsules) every eight hours.
- **Naproxen sodium** (Aleve). Take 500 mg (two 250-mg tablets) every 12 hours.
- **Acetaminophen** (Tylenol, others). Take 1,000 mg (two 500-mg tablets) every six hours.

Sometimes you need to jiggle the clots quite briskly to get them to dissolve. Don't worry, you won't damage any tissue as you do this. If there's only blood in the strainer, simply rinse the strainer and have it near the toilet for the next time you use the bathroom.

At some point, you'll see tissue within the clots — it often appears tan or gray. This tissue is a combination of the pregnancy sac and of the lining of your uterus (decidua). Some people say the sac looks like a cotton ball in water. It can be hard to tell the difference without using medical equipment. If your pregnancy is 10 weeks or older, you may see the baby itself within the tissue. (Rarely, you can see the baby if you're eight or nine weeks along).

You can place any tissue you collect into the jar or cup with a lid. If you have saline solution, you can pour a little into the container to keep the tissue damp. When the bleeding slows and you think you've passed all the pregnancy tissue, you can put the container in a bag inside your refrigerator until you're ready to bring the tissue into the doctor's office for testing.

It's safe to take acetaminophen with either ibuprofen *or* naproxen, but *do not* take ibuprofen and naproxen together or even on the same day. Also, do not take aspirin during this time. It will thin your blood and may make your bleeding heavier.

WHEN IT'S OVER

Most of my patients tell me they know the miscarriage is over because it's "like a storm passed." They feel physically much better, in terms of both cramping and bleeding. For other people, the change is more gradual, and they feel a little better each day over multiple days.

But some people get tired of waiting for it to be over. It's not uncommon for people to choose to wait out the miscarriage, but then call my office after a week or two and ask how much longer they need to wait.

Do I ever have to stop waiting?

Most miscarriages begin within two weeks of diagnosis, but it can take up to eight weeks before bleeding begins. The risk of infection is incredibly low, even if it seems to take forever to begin the process. So, there's no need to change your plan. If you're feeling well — no severe cramping, no fever — there's no real need for surgery or medical treatment. Doctors know that 80% of people will have a complete miscarriage within eight weeks of waiting, but it's unclear what your chances of success are if you're waiting longer than that. That said, you can always decide that enough is enough and ask for a more active management of the miscarriage.

However, if your pregnancy is over 10 weeks along, you're more likely to need medication or surgery to complete the miscarriage, even if you do choose expectant management. Talk to your doctor about what options might be best for you.

Your doctor will want to make sure that you've passed the entire pregnancy, so it's wise to have a follow-up visit after the miscarriage is over. I schedule my patients for a visit 2 to 7 days after they think the miscarriage has completed. Some doctors will perform an ultrasound to look inside your uterus, while others will perform a gentle physical exam to see if your cervix is still open and to make sure you're not having any tenderness in your uterus.

If you prefer to not go into the office for follow-up, your doctor or a nurse can speak with you on the phone about your symptoms. If your bleeding and cramping were heavy but are now better, and you're not feeling any further pregnancy symptoms, this can indicate that your miscarriage is over.

POTENTIAL COMPLICATIONS

I said in the last chapter that all methods of miscarriage management are safe, and that's true. There are a few possible complications, though, no matter which path you choose. Here's a brief look at each of these possible complications.

Heavy bleeding

Bleeding is a risk during miscarriage care, no matter which treatment you choose. The longer it takes for your body to pass the pregnancy, the higher the risk of overly heavy bleeding.

Infection

The risk of infection is the lowest with expectant management, but it's still present. Just like with the risk of heavy bleeding, the more time that passes between your diagnosis and your miscarriage, the greater the risk of infection.

Failure to pass the pregnancy

Doctors know that waiting it out works for most people. But we don't have good information about what the chances of success are for people who still haven't passed their pregnancy after eight weeks. And this doesn't mean eight weeks since you first found out you were having a miscarriage — that's eight weeks after the end of the pregnancy.

For instance, at the time of your 12-week ultrasound, you may have found out that the embryo was only eight weeks in size, meaning the pregnancy stopped growing four weeks before. In this case, even though you just found out about the loss, your body has already begun the process of waiting out the miscarriage. And if you decide to manage the loss expectantly, after another four weeks pass, it will really be eight weeks from the time the pregnancy stopped.

Warning signs to watch for

Your doctor will likely give you a list of warning signs to look out for when you're waiting for the miscarriage to start. I tell my patients to call my office if any of the following happens:

- **The pain is too severe.** The cramps with a miscarriage are no joke, and most people need to take pain medication (see "Managing pain" on page 68). But if you're taking the maximum doses of pain medication and it's not relieving your pain, don't suffer in silence. Call your doctor.
- **The bleeding is too heavy.** During the most intense part of the miscarriage, you may bleed heavier than your usual period, including blood clots up to the size of a pingpong ball. But if you're filling a maxi pad end-to-end in an hour for two straight hours or passing bigger blood clots the size of an egg or larger, let your doctor know.
- **You feel dizzy.** If you're having heavy bleeding and you start to feel dizzy when you're walking or even just sitting

up, it may be a sign that you're losing too much blood too quickly. Call your doctor.

- **You have a fever.** Getting an infection during the process of a miscarriage is very unusual, but it can happen. If you have a temperature of over 100.4 F (38 C), call your doctor.

✓ QUESTIONS TO ASK YOUR DOCTOR

Bring this list of questions to your appointment to ask regarding expectant management for treatment of your miscarriage. Take notes and check off the questions as you go.

☐ How long do you think it might take my body to start the miscarriage if I don't do anything to help it along?

_____

☐ If I want to wait out the miscarriage, how can I follow up with questions?

_____

☐ How long do you think it's safe for me to wait to see if the miscarriage starts on its own?

_____

☐ When should I come back to the office for a visit?

_____

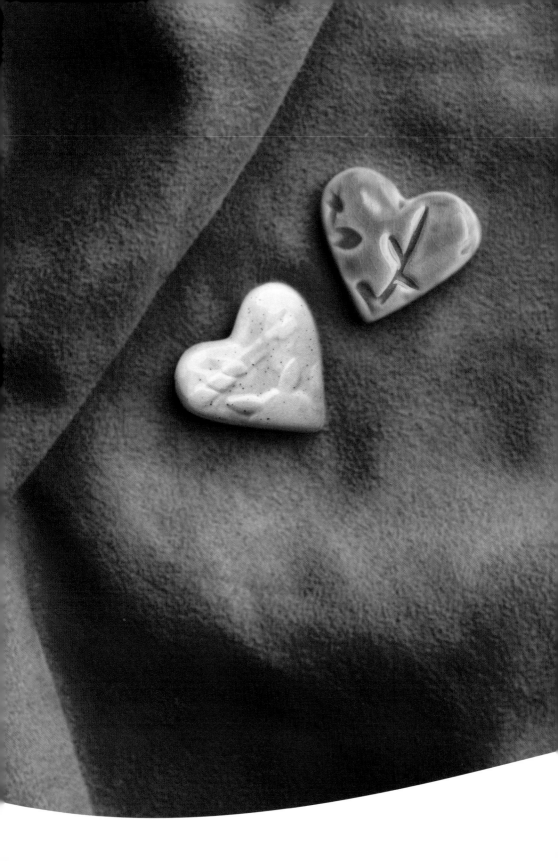

CHAPTER 5

Medical management: Get it going

Evelyn waited for me while sitting on the exam table, arms crossed. Her third visit in the past two weeks, she was "waiting for her miscarriage to happen naturally" — but she had yet to start bleeding. "I'm tired of this," Evelyn told me. I offered her a surgical procedure at the end of the week, but she adamantly declined. "What else can we do?" she asked.

Medical management of a first trimester miscarriage is the middle ground between waiting for nature to take its course and scheduling a procedure. Some people don't want to wait for the pregnancy to pass on its own — it's the least invasive treatment, but also the most unpredictable path and might take the longest amount of time. Others hesitate to undergo surgery. With surgery, you know exactly when it's going to happen, but it carries some risks.

For these people, medication management is an ideal choice. Medication kick-starts the natural process of your body passing the pregnancy tissue. Doctors can do this when your body has determined that the pregnancy is no longer progressing, but your body hasn't yet begun to expel the pregnancy from your uterus.

HOW MEDICAL MANAGEMENT WORKS

Doctors mainly use two medications to manage a miscarriage:
1. **Mifepristone,** which is often called by its nickname, mife (pronounced MIF-ee), and may also be referred to by its brand name, Mifeprex.
2. **Misoprostol,** which is often called by its nickname, miso (pronounced MEE-so), and may also be referred to by its brand name, Cytotec. More casually online and elsewhere, it's referred to as the "star pill" because of its hexagonal shape.

In this book, I refer to them by their nicknames, mife and miso, because it's what doctors use (plus, they're much easier to say). You'll likely take both medications in the course of your miscarriage. That's because they work together, increasing your chance of successfully completing your miscarriage without needing a surgical procedure.

But not all doctors' offices and hospitals have mife available to give patients, and it's not a medication that you can get by prescription. If your doctor doesn't mention mife, you can ask if that's an option for you. While not quite as effective on its own, most of the time miso alone works to complete the miscarriage if mifepristone isn't available.

Using medication gives you a private experience for your miscarriage in the comfort of your own home, rather than in your doctor's office or a hospital. You'll want to make some preparations before you take the miso, however, because bleeding and cramping can last for hours, and it can be unpredictable.

Just as you would when you are suffering from a GI bug or on a horrible period day, put on your most comfortable clothes and curl up at home, although not necessarily in bed. I don't advise staying in bed because you can't help but focus on the pain you're experiencing. Find something that can distract you, whether it's binge-watching a show on Netflix, scrolling through your Facebook feed, talking to a friend on the phone, listening to music or falling down the Pinterest rabbit hole and

THE OTHER 'M' MEDICATION

While misoprostol is the best choice for kick-starting a miscarriage, if yours has already started, then your doctor may give you methylergonovine (Methergine) instead of miso. Methergine has fewer side effects than miso, but it's only effective if the body has passed some of the pregnancy tissue but not all of it. Your doctor might also give you Methergine if you experience very heavy bleeding after taking miso or after having a procedure, as it is good at slowing the bleeding down.

trying to craft something — whatever will be soothing for you. I also recommend comfort food, although nausea can be a side effect of the medication.

If your doctor has given you any prescriptions for pain medication, or you need to refill your own stock of acetaminophen (Tylenol, others) and ibuprofen (Advil, Motrin IB, others) or naproxen sodium (Aleve), make sure you go to the drugstore before taking the miso. That way you have the medications on hand if you need them.

I'm a big believer in using pain medication *before* you start feeling any pain. As soon as you take the miso — or even just before — start taking an anti-inflammatory pain medication. Take it around the clock, as directed on the label, for the first day or two. That way you're never chasing the pain. Once the pain starts to get intense, it takes a lot more medication to get it under control.

Internet alert

If you search online for miso and mife — a bad idea because the information you find could be confusing — you may see three things about them that are important to understand. Here's what you need to know.

First: Miso was originally developed to protect people from developing stomach ulcers when they routinely use anti-inflammatory drugs. It's amazing that a drug developed for a completely different reason can treat people with miscarriages. But in reality, many drugs are routinely used for more than one purpose. For example, did you know that minoxidil (Rogaine) was originally developed as a drug to treat high blood pressure? So, don't think that your doctor is confused and is treating you for the wrong conditions or with the wrong medication! I consider miso a magical drug with many purposes.

Second: You might find that miso is not recommended (contraindicated) in pregnancy. You may see warnings that pregnant people shouldn't use this medication. The reason for these warnings is that taking miso during a healthy pregnancy puts the fetus at risk of certain serious birth defects. So, that warning is true for people who are continuing a healthy pregnancy. But since you're facing a miscarriage, there's no reason to be concerned.

Finally: You might read that these medications are also used as the regimen for an abortion. This is true. Mife and miso are used for both clinical situations — for people who are having an abortion to end a pregnancy, as well as for people who want to accelerate the passing of a pregnancy that has already been lost due to miscarriage. But just because you're given these medications doesn't mean that you're having an abortion, which is the ending of a healthy pregnancy. Your pregnancy is over, so mife and miso are just helping your miscarriage end more quickly.

Taking mife

If your doctor uses mife as part of the treatment for miscarriage, you'll take this medication first. You can even take it on the same day you decide to proceed with medical management. The dose of mife is 200 milligrams (mg) in a single tablet that you'll swallow in front of your doctor. Many of my patients begin having light to moderate bleeding hours after taking mife. Some feel nothing, and some report heavy bleeding later that evening.

Regardless of the impact, it's important to take the miso tablets as well, as directed by your doctor. These two medications work together to complete your miscarriage. Mife, when taken on its own, will not reliably cause your uterus to pass all the pregnancy tissue.

Taking miso

If you took mife, you'll take miso roughly 24 to 36 hours later, and no more than 72 hours later. We don't know if miso will still be effective if you take it outside of this time window. However, if you're only taking miso, you have some flexibility.

I talk to my patients about timing the medication around what's convenient for them. You'll most likely start bleeding and cramping within 3 to 4 hours after you take miso, but bleeding may begin as quickly as 30 minutes after. For some people, it takes up to a day before they start bleeding. This unpredictability is one of the downsides of this approach.

Here are some steps you can take to make the process go more smoothly:

- Fill your pain medication prescriptions at the pharmacy, or make sure you have plenty of anti-inflammatories at the ready in your medicine cabinet (ibuprofen, naproxen and acetaminophen).
- Take a dose of ibuprofen or naproxen before you take the miso tablets.
- Make sure you can be in a comfortable, safe place when you take the miso — somewhere with easy access to a bathroom.
- Wear comfy clothes. They may will help you feel better when the cramping begins.
- Plan to eat a light meal that day, and drink as much fluid as you want to (though maybe not alcohol).
- Plan some distractions for yourself, whether it's TV, the internet, a new book or something else.
- If you have kiddos at home, consider arranging child care so that you can focus on your own physical needs.

Consider waiting until you've done some errands or finished the things you need to do that day, because once the bleeding and cramping start, you're going to want to be home, near your own bathroom. The absolute *worst* time to take miso is when you're going to be out and about. I also wouldn't recommend taking it at bedtime. It's a surefire way to ruin a good night's sleep.

Regardless of whether you've taken mife or not, the way to take miso is the same. The most common dose is 800 micrograms. The largest-sized tablet for miso is 200 micrograms, which means that you'll likely get four separate tablets from your doctor. You may get the medication in the office, in an envelope or a bottle, or you may receive a prescription to fill at a pharmacy.

The most important thing to remember: Don't swallow them! The tablets still work if you swallow them, but they'll likely make you extremely nauseous. The better way to take the pills is buccally — by placing the tablets in your mouth, between your cheek and your gums, and letting them dissolve there. It's in the same place that baseball players tuck their chewing tobacco when you see them in the dugout. It may feel like a strange way to take medicine, but it gets the medication into your bloodstream faster and bypasses your stomach, which lowers your risk of nausea and vomiting.

My patients tell me the miso tablets have a chalky taste, but they're not bitter. One of my patients said, "It's like sucking on paper." If there is any pill residue left after 30 minutes, it's safe to swallow it — at this point, the medication has been absorbed and all that's left is the starchy coating of the pill. Do not eat and drink while the pills are in place in your cheeks, since that's likely to wash them down into your stomach. But it's fine to eat both before and after you take the tablets.

The other, even stranger, place to put the miso tablets is directly into your vagina. Believe it or not, the vagina is a great way to take medication. Miso can be completely absorbed this way, won't give you a funny taste in your mouth and avoids the risk of it upsetting your stomach. If you're not having heavy bleeding from your miscarriage, this may be an ideal way to take them.

To go this route, use the bathroom first — you don't want to have to pee after you place the pills and risk them falling into the toilet. Then, place the pills, one at a time, high up in your vagina (as high as you can easily reach) so that they don't fall out if you cough or laugh. If you feel too dry, and the pills are getting stuck on the way in, you can use a tiny amount of lubricant on your finger to make it easier. But don't let the pills get too coated in lube or they'll have a hard time dissolving.

You don't have to worry about taking miso with other medications, like those for allergies, asthma, high blood pressure or

depression. There are no contrain-
dications or interactions between
miso and other commonly used
medications, either prescription or
over the counter.

> **Is it OK if I'm taking other medications when I take miso?**

DURING THE MISCARRIAGE

When you take miso, the bleeding can be very heavy at first, so

MEDICATIONS AT A GLANCE		
Medication	**When to take it**	**How to take it**
Mifepristone (mife)	In the doctor's office, once you've decided on medical management	By mouth, with some water
Pain medication	Right before taking the miso tablets	By mouth, with some water
Misoprostol (miso)	24 to 72 hours after swallowing the mife; or, if you're not taking mife, then as soon as it's convenient for you (not recommended right before bed)	Buccally, between your gums and your cheeks; alternatively, place the tablets in your vagina

heavy that you might even be soaking a whole maxi pad in an hour for a couple of hours straight. You also might pass blood clots that are much larger than you have with your periods, with some as big as pingpong balls. You may or may not see tissue or the pregnancy sac pass with the blood clots.

While the worst of the bleeding and cramping often lasts for 1 to 2 days, the total duration of bleeding with a miscarriage lasts much longer than a typical period — on and off for up to three weeks. It sucks, but it's normal.

Besides bleeding, you can count on cramping pain. To ease the pain, I recommend stocking up on your favorite anti-inflammatories, whether it's ibuprofen, naproxen or acetaminophen. (See "Managing pain" on page 68 for the best way to dose over-the-counter pain medications.) You can also ask your doctor for a prescription for higher strength ibuprofen or naproxen. They'll be bigger tablets that might be harder to swallow, but you get to take them less often.

Here's the secret to maximizing over-the-counter pain relief. The trick is to use a combination of pain medicines. Ibuprofen and naproxen sodium are in the same category of pain medication, which means you shouldn't take them at the same time. Pick your favorite and stick with that one and take it as your doctor recommends. Acetaminophen works in a different way, so you can use it along with ibuprofen or naproxen.

I tell patients to alternate these medications, taking the ibuprofen or naproxen first, then taking acetaminophen 2 to 3 hours later, and then repeating the cycle. That way, you're never too far from your next dose of pain medication.

I don't want to scare you with how this sounds. Not everyone experiences incredibly bad pain, but some people do. I'd rather prepare you for the worst. That way you're not concerned if it happens — and then if it's better than this, that's wonderful.

You may also experience flu-like signs and symptoms like vomiting, diarrhea, a low-grade fever and chills. The symptoms usually last less than a day, but if you have severe nausea or vomiting, ask your doctor for a prescription for medication.

WHEN IT'S OVER

In most cases, after several hours of heavy bleeding and cramping, you start to feel better. Your bleeding flow should lighten, and cramps should become less intense. Many patients have told me after this process that they knew the medication worked because there was a distinct change in how they were feeling — they didn't need pain medication anymore and weren't going to the bathroom to change their pads as often.

People worry that they're going to see something upsetting or recognizable when they start bleeding. You won't always be able to tell when the pregnancy is passing — for many people, the tissue itself is hidden within blood clots, or passes directly into the toilet. Let me reassure you: The bleeding is

What do I do when I see the pregnancy pass?

going to look just like a heavy period. If you are nine weeks along in your pregnancy or earlier, it's unlikely you're going to see anything that looks like a baby come out of your body. You know how sometimes when you're on your period, you might see something gray and tissue-like amidst the blood clots. That's a little bit of the lining of your uterus coming out. You might see something similar with a miscarriage, but you likely won't see anything that's going to make you feel sad.

If you are further along in the first trimester (10 to 12 weeks), there is a moderate chance that you will see the baby. If this prospect is unacceptable to you, talk with your doctor about other treatment options.

For early miscarriages, most people simply flush the tissue along with the bleeding. If this approach feels wrong to you, there is another option. When the doctor gives you the prescription for misoprostol, ask for a specimen cup. It looks like the kind you pee into when you give a urine sample. Use the cup to scoop up the pregnancy tissue, then you can bury it or bring it to your doctor's office. Some doctors may offer the specimen cup to you for this purpose, but in my experience, it's more common to need to ask your doctor. Read about this process in detail in Chapter 4. Your doctor can send the tissue for examination that can include looking for infection and performing genetic testing.

The best way to know for sure that the miscarriage is over is to go back to your doctor's office for follow-up. Your doctor may want you to come in 2 to 3 days after you start bleeding or may wait as long as a week to give your body the maximum chance to pass the pregnancy. At this visit, you'll likely have an exam or a transvaginal ultrasound exam to make sure that your uterus is empty and that you don't have any remaining large blood clots or tissue left inside. Once your doctor gives you the all-clear based on the exam and the ultrasound, you know the miscarriage is finished. If you can't get back in for follow-up, have a telemedicine visit to discuss your symptoms.

IF THE MEDICATION DOESN'T WORK

Some people don't have much bleeding after one dose of miso. They only have a little bit of spotting, or maybe even no bleeding at all. In some cases, even with bleeding or cramping like I describe, the ultrasound shows that there's still tissue inside the uterus. If that's the case, the miscarriage is not yet over. The next step can be another dose of miso, scheduling a procedure or waiting things out. If you're not having heavy bleeding or severe pain, you'll have all three of your original options available to you again.

For patients who want to continue medical management of their miscarriage, I offer a second dose of miso that they can take 1 to 3 days after the first dose. Your doctor may also offer you a second dose and give you up to a week to take it. Sometimes the second jolt gets things started. I'll then ask them to follow up in about a week for another ultrasound to confirm that their uterus is empty.

Sometimes people have a rough experience with the pills and don't want to use them again, especially if they had severe chills or diarrhea. In this case, if you prefer, you can go to expectant management. There's no rule that says you must have more miso, or that you must have surgery. If you're not showing any signs of infection or hemorrhage, there's no reason that you can't just wait a little bit longer for your body to finish the miscarriage, if that's the approach you'd like to take.

POTENTIAL COMPLICATIONS

There are very few risks to completing a miscarriage with medication. The biggest thing to look out for is incredibly heavy bleeding. I tell my patients to call me right away if they're filling a pad end-to-end with blood in an hour for more than two hours straight, passing blood clots the size of an egg or larger, or passing continuous clots. Your doctor may want you to come in to either have extra medical therapy, or in rare cases, an emergency surgery (dilation and curettage) to finish the miscarriage so that you stop bleeding.

Another potential complication is severe pain. Pain levels are different for everybody, and we all experience pain in different ways. But if you know that you have a hard time with severe menstrual cramps or other pain, definitely talk to your doctor about a prescription for pain medication to get you through the worst of the miscarriage. And if all the pain medications you have aren't working, please call your doctor.

Warning signs to watch for

Your doctor will likely give you a list of warning signs to look out for when using medication to manage a miscarriage. I tell my patients to call my office if any of the following happens:

- **The pain is too severe.** Refer to "Managing pain" on page 68 for pain medications and doses that work for miscarriage. If the maximum doses aren't relieving your pain, call your doctor's office.
- **The bleeding is too heavy.** During the most intense part of the miscarriage, you may bleed more heavily than you

---

✓ QUESTIONS TO ASK YOUR DOCTOR

Bring this list of questions to your appointment when you discuss options for medication management of your miscarriage. Take notes and check off the questions as you go.

☐ If I want to use medical management, what medications do you prescribe?

_____

_____

☐ If miso is one of the medications, do you recommend taking it vaginally or buccally?

_____

☐ Can you show me how to take the miso?

_____

---

would during a regular period, and pass blood clots as big as a pingpong ball. But if you're filling a maxi pad end-to-end in an hour for two straight hours or passing blood clots the size of an egg, your doctor wants to know about it.

- **You feel dizzy.** If you're having heavy bleeding and you start to feel dizzy when you're walking or even sitting up, it may be a sign that you're losing too much blood too quickly.
- **You're feeling sick for more than a day.** Call your doctor if your nausea, vomiting, diarrhea or fever lasts for more than 24 hours after taking misoprostol — these could be signs and symptoms of infection.

☐ Do you have mifepristone in your office? If you don't have mifepristone, is there another office you can refer me to?

_____

☐ Should I schedule a follow-up appointment, or should I call when I think I passed the pregnancy?

_____

☐ If I want to have the pregnancy tissue examined or tested, can you give me a specimen cup so that I can try to bring the tissue into the office?

_____

☐ I don't want to flush the pregnancy tissue. Can I get a specimen cup to collect it?

_____

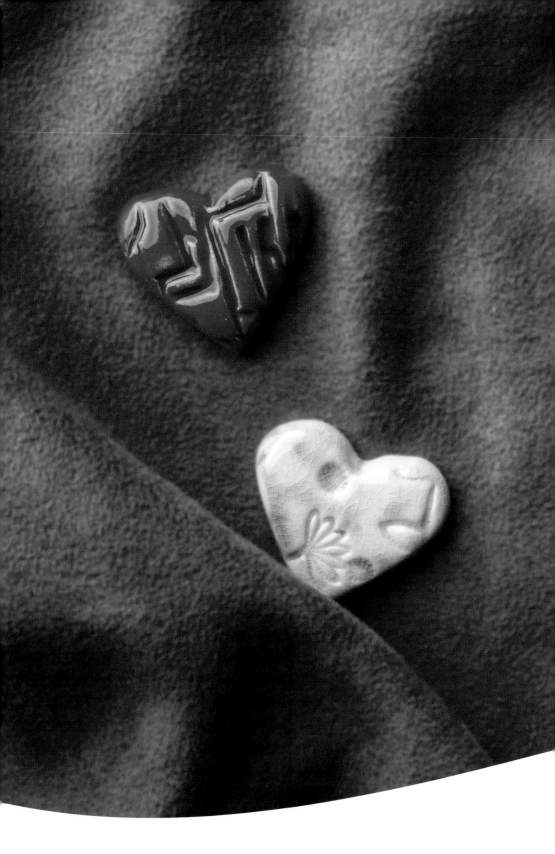

CHAPTER 6

Surgical management: Just getting it done

Our clinic received a call from the ultrasound unit. Fiona had just had her 11-week genetic screening ultrasound, and she was diagnosed with a miscarriage. Her baby had stopped growing at eight weeks, but she had had no cramping or bleeding at all.

Fiona walked with her partner over to our side of the clinic. Through tears, she told us she wanted to have a procedure as soon as possible. She said, "I can't stand the thought of carrying a dead baby around inside of me any longer."

For people who just want their first trimester miscarriage over and done with as soon as possible, or for those who aren't comfortable waiting once they know the pregnancy is over, a surgical procedure is the ideal choice.

The word *surgery* may sound daunting, especially if you're a person who never had your tonsils or your appendix out. But surgery is a big umbrella term for any kind of procedure that involves entering the body. Essentially, a straightforward, five-minute procedure for a miscarriage that doesn't involve any incisions gets the same shorthand label as brain surgery or a kidney transplant.

HAVING A D&C

First, let's talk about what the procedure is. When your body is having a miscarriage, the safest way to end the pregnancy with a surgical procedure is to place instruments into the vagina, through your cervix, and into your uterus to remove the pregnancy tissue. This process is called a dilation and curettage (D&C). You first learned about this procedure in Chapter 3.

The procedure gets this name from the two major parts of the procedure: The D refers to the dilation of the cervix, and the C refers to the removal of the pregnancy by scraping or scooping

---

(i) MEDICINE-TO-ENGLISH TRANSLATION

These basic terms will be helpful for you to understand as you read through this chapter.

Dilation and curettage (D&C). A two-step procedure of stretching open the natural opening of your cervix with dilators, then removing the pregnancy, typically with suction, rather than a scraping with a metal instrument (curetting). Also called vacuum or suction aspiration or suction curettage.

Electric aspiration. Use of an electric vacuum pump to remove the pregnancy tissue from the uterus. Most often used in a procedure or operating room, though can also be used in the office.

Intravenous (IV). Placing a tiny, plastic tube (catheter) into a vein in your hand or your arm. Allows the nurse or doctor to give you fluids and medications to help make the procedure more comfortable.

(curettage). Today, most doctors use vacuum aspiration, not scraping, so the name *D&C* isn't exactly medically accurate anymore, but it's how most people still refer to this surgery. You may also hear your doctor call it a "suction curettage" or an "aspiration procedure."

If your pregnancy is later in the first trimester — around 12 or 13 weeks — your doctor may want to give you a medication before surgery. This is called misoprostol (Cytotec), which I

My doctor wants to give me medication — but I thought I was getting a procedure?

Local anesthesia. Injection of a numbing medication into your vagina around your cervix. Sounds much worse than it feels.

Manual vacuum aspiration. Use of a hand-held, hand-activated large plastic syringe to remove the pregnancy tissue from the uterus. Looks like a turkey baster (see page 96).

Paracervical block. Injection of a numbing medication (anesthetic) through the wall of the vagina around the cervix. Causes a cramping sensation when the medication goes in. Doesn't take all of the procedure pain away, but makes it more comfortable.

Vacuum aspiration. Another — more accurate — name for a dilation and curettage (D&C) procedure, since it's rare for an actual "curettage" with a metal scraping instrument to take place. Removes the contents of the uterus through a plastic or metal cannula, attached to a vacuum source.

talked about in Chapter 5. You use a smaller dose (400 micrograms) 2 to 3 hours before surgery to soften your cervix and make it easier to dilate during the procedure. While you may have some side effects like nausea, cramping or diarrhea, overall, this medication may make the procedure safer and faster.

A D&C involves a few steps. The first step feels like the Pap test you have during your annual OB-GYN exam, since it involves putting a speculum into your vagina. Your doctor then cleans your cervix and your vagina with soap, which might feel cold and a little pokey, but not painful.

Then you'll be given local anesthesia called lidocaine. This is what your dentist gives you when you're getting a cavity filled. Your doctor injects the lidocaine around your cervix; this is called a paracervical block. While this may sound horrible, the injections actually feel more like menstrual cramps. Not pleasant, but not fully unfamiliar. After the injections, you won't feel completely numb, like having an epidural, but the sensations of the procedure will be dulled, and you'll feel more

WHY A PARACERVICAL BLOCK ISN'T EXCRUCIATINGLY PAINFUL

Need more reassurance that injections of lidocaine around your cervix won't hurt much? The skin in the vagina doesn't have nearly the number of nerve endings that you have in your mouth where your dentist gives you lidocaine injections. This explains why many women can't have an orgasm from intercourse alone — the nerves that detect feel-good sensations just aren't there. That's why the vaginal injections don't feel sharp. Not a great situation for sex, but it's reassuring when it comes to procedures.

cramping than sharp pain. Then your doctor stretches open (dilates) the natural opening of your cervix.

Some of my patients worry that they're going to be cut open somehow, because they think of surgery as involving scalpels. And the word *curettage* even sounds like it has the word *cut* when you say it quickly. But your cervix already has an opening. It's not only how sperm got into your uterus to get you pregnant, but it's how menstrual blood from your uterus flows into your vagina every month. We can use that natural opening and just stretch it a bit using metal or plastic instruments called dilators. No incisions at all. Dilating often causes a sensation more like an achy pressure than sharp pain.

Once your cervix is sufficiently opened, your doctor places a narrow plastic tube that looks like a thick soda straw into your uterus. This tube, called a curette, is then attached to a vacuum device that removes the pregnancy (see page 96).

There are two ways that pregnancy tissue can be removed when you're having an early miscarriage. The traditional method is called electric aspiration, where your doctor uses a machine with a motor that makes a low-pitched mechanical noise during the procedure. But it doesn't sound like any other vacuum cleaner you've likely used in your life. So, you won't flash back to the procedure the next time you clean your home. And there's no funky smell, like you may notice when getting a tooth drilled.

The other technique is manual vacuum aspiration, sometimes called an MVA. For this method, your doctor uses a hand-held device that looks like a turkey baster to create a vacuum that takes the pregnancy out. For pregnancies under nine weeks, this can be a quieter alternative to using the electric vacuum. Both procedures are safe. And honestly, they both hurt about the same amount. Your doctor typically explains which technique will be used, and you can talk about it beforehand.

WHAT AN MVA LOOKS LIKE

A manual vacuum aspirator (MVA) (A) is a hand-held device used to remove a pregnancy. A curette, which comes in different sizes (B and C), is attached to the MVA.

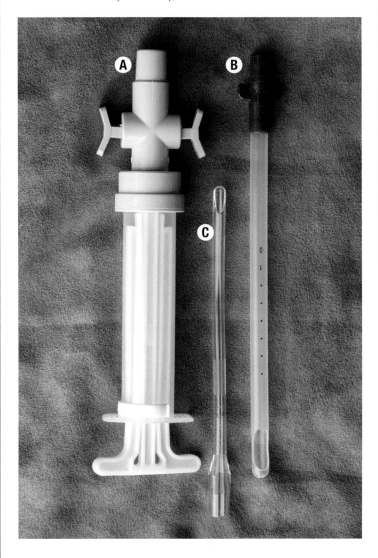

For many people, suction is the most intense part. It feels like menstrual cramps, but more severe. You can think of this as the worst period pain you've had in your life. The cramping can peak right at the end of the procedure. Once your uterus realizes that it's empty, it's going to clamp down very quickly, like it's forming a fist. This reaction is actually a good thing because it prevents you from bleeding too much at the end of the procedure. But this contracting can feel intense.

The good news is that this suction part usually takes about 90 seconds for most miscarriages. *Just 90 seconds?* you might think. *That's so fast!* Yes, this whole procedure start to finish — from the speculum going in until the last instruments come out — is typically under seven minutes. Sometimes under five.

After your doctor takes all the instruments out, you have time to recover. In as little as 30 minutes after the procedure, you'll feel pretty much like your usual self when you're having your period. You'll walk out of the office or hospital on your own, and you won't be hunched over or need a wheelchair to get to your car. That doesn't mean that your heart may not be hurting, but at least your body will be feeling close to normal.

PROCEDURE OPTIONS

Depending on how your doctor practices and whether procedures are performed in an office, a surgical suite or an operating room, you may have different options for anesthesia. Here's what to expect with the most common options.

In an office

The simplest way to have the procedure for a miscarriage is to have it right in your doctor's office, in the same place where you get your birth control and you have your Pap tests. Not all doctor's offices are set up for procedures, though, so this might not be an option for you. In most cases, the only anesthesia available in an office is local anesthesia, which is just the injection around your cervix alone. Your doctor may also be able to give you oral medication for pain and for anxiety.

In a surgical suite

A surgical suite is not a full-fledged operating room, but it has more equipment and more options than a typical doctor's office. This is the setup of most Planned Parenthood clinics. In these facilities, there are separate procedure rooms and recovery rooms, and you're often able to have an IV placed into your hand or arm, so you can receive medications that help with both anxiety and pain. This option is often referred to as IV moderate sedation or conscious sedation. Having this level of medication makes you sleepy during the procedure. Most people don't fall completely asleep, but almost everyone is more relaxed and more comfortable than if they just had local lidocaine injections.

To have these IV medications, you'll need to have a completely empty stomach, which means you can't eat anything for eight hours before the procedure. Some doctors also insist that you not drink anything after midnight the night before, while others allow you to have clear liquids (water, clear broth) up until two hours before the procedure. Check with your doctor for specifics. You'll also need to have someone drive you home. (No, an Uber or Lyft doesn't count.)

In an operating room

The ultimate comfort for some people is to go to an operating room in a hospital. This approach allows them to have a much deeper level of sedation, which is called deep anesthesia or sometimes general anesthesia. When you get "general," a tube is placed down your throat once you're fully asleep, and your breathing is controlled by an anesthesiologist during the procedure. It may feel like a big production for such a quick procedure, but for people who are afraid of pain or are simply terrified of being awake during a procedure, they may elect the operating room option.

Sometimes it takes longer to schedule these procedures. Operating rooms are busy and not user-friendly when it comes to nonemergency procedures. (What feels like an emergency to you may not be deemed an emergency by the hospital.) You may not be able to have a procedure in an operating room as quickly as you'd like, but for many people, this is an option.

(?) YOU MAY BE THINKING …

Can I have my partner or a friend with me during the procedure?

Every doctor's office is different, but in general, you can have your partner or a support person with you during a procedure in an office under local anesthesia. If you're having a procedure in a surgical suite or operating room, you may be able to have someone with you while you're waiting, but you likely won't be able to have someone with you in the procedure room.

If you're having your procedure in a place where there are other patients waiting for procedures in the same room, it's possible that your partner will need to wait in the waiting room until your procedure is finished. While it may seem like a cruel policy, it's to protect the privacy of the other patients who are there.

WHEN IT'S OVER

Unlike waiting it out with expectant management or using medication for your miscarriage with medical management, a surgical procedure lets your doctor know right away when they've removed the whole pregnancy by examining the removed tissue. Right after the procedure, the doctor examines the pregnancy tissue to confirm that all the tissue was removed from your uterus. We can tell based on the size of the pregnancy sac that we've gotten the whole thing.

After this examination, the pathology department often examines and confirms the findings. Genetic testing on the tissue would be performed at this point. In most cases, the pregnancy tissue — the pregnancy sac, placental tissue, and the embryo or fetus, if present — are then cremated, but not in a way that you can receive ashes afterwards. If a burial or receiving ashes is important to you, you can work with a funeral home to take the baby from the hospital after testing. State regulations vary, but it's rare that you're allowed to take the pregnancy tissue home yourself after a D&C.

On the day of the procedure and the days that follow, you should have a level of bleeding and cramping that are like your period. Bleeding should not be heavier than the heaviest day of your period, whatever that means for you. This means that passing a small clot the size of a quarter might be OK but passing multiple large blood clots (as big as an egg) is not. If you have heavier bleeding than you normally experience with a period, call your doctor.

Bleeding can last up to two weeks after the procedure. It won't be period-heavy the entire time — most of my patients have either period-like bleeding that gradually tapers off, or on-and-off random bleeding. If I see my patients for a two-week post-procedure check, most of them are either having mild spotting or no bleeding at all.

Less common is when people have *no* bleeding after the procedure. After being counseled to expect all that bleeding, it can freak you out to see nothing on your pad. If you're not feeling intense cramping, though, it's totally fine to not bleed. You'll likely start bleeding in a few days. But if you do have worsening pain when you're home, make sure to call your doctor.

For tampon and menstrual cup fans, I regret to inform you that it's better to use pads during this time. There is a slight risk of infection after the procedure, so you want the blood to be able to flow easily and completely out of your body. However, period underwear like Thinx is totally fine once the heaviest of the bleeding has passed.

Cramps are the most intense in the first two days after the procedure, so have anti-inflammatories around and take as much as you need to for those days. You may want to take them on and off for a week afterwards when you have cramps some days but not others. Overall, you should feel less pain with each passing day.

If you had any kind of IV anesthesia, expect to feel a little odd for a day or two afterward. You may feel completely fine as you leave the hospital, and then start to feel wonky a few hours later. This is expected. It usually takes a day or two for the drugs to completely leave your system, so don't make any big decisions — like a dramatic haircut or a job change — in these two days after getting anesthesia. You might feel like doing nothing more than hopping into bed and going to sleep, and if that's what your body is telling you to do, then do it.

After an uncomplicated procedure, you don't have to follow up at the doctor's office. But if you feel better going back to the doctor for a check just to make sure that you're OK, make an appointment for about two weeks after the procedure. Much of the bleeding should be over at that point, the pain should be gone, and you should be feeling physically back to normal.

If you do have complications, they are going to make themselves known: Too much pain, too much bleeding or a fever. If this is the case, call your doctor. But you won't have any hidden complications. If you're feeling good, I tell my patients, then you are good.

Potential complications

It's important to know that having a D&C for a miscarriage is incredibly safe. In fact, it's much safer than having a baby. That said, there is a less than 1% risk of developing one of the following conditions, which your doctor will discuss with you.

Heavy bleeding during the procedure Every time a pregnancy ends — whether with delivery or miscarriage — there's a risk of excessive bleeding. Most of the time, this bleeding can be controlled with medications. On rare occasions, more-intensive procedures are required to stop your bleeding.

Heavy bleeding at home You should expect bleeding like a period, on and off but eventually tapering, for about two weeks. So heavier bleeding than this — passing large (egg-sized) clots or soaking through more than one maxi pad in an hour — requires medical attention.

Infection You'll likely receive antibiotics around the time of the procedure, which makes the risk of infection in your uterus very small. But if you experience fever or chills, severe pelvic pain, or see an unusual yellow or green vaginal discharge, you need to call your doctor.

Perforation Rarely, a surgical instrument can create a small hole in the uterus. Often, this heals on its own and only requires watchful waiting and a follow-up exam. But sometimes additional surgery is required to confirm that nothing in your abdomen was injured or to repair an injury if there is one.

Retained tissue Your doctor can confirm that the procedure is complete in two ways: First, the inside of your uterus has a distinct feel with the instruments when all the tissue has been removed; and second, through direct examination of the tissue. Your doctor may want to perform an ultrasound exam in the procedure room if he or she isn't sure the procedure is complete. But your body still needs to pass small amounts of uterine lining (decidua) and blood clots after the procedure — it's why it's not uncommon to bleed for a week or two.

Very heavy bleeding or no bleeding at all, along with cramps that don't get better with time, might mean you have retained tissue that needs to be removed with an additional D&C.

As scary as all these things sound, it's important to put the risks into perspective. Statistically speaking, the riskiest part of the procedure is the drive to the doctor's office. You can feel secure knowing that this is a safe option, if it's the one that best meets your needs.

Warning signs to watch for

Your doctor should give you a list of warning signs to look out for after your D&C. I tell my patients to call my office if:

- **Their pain is too severe.** I've listed medications and doses that work for miscarriage in Chapter 4. But if the maximum doses aren't relieving your pain, call your doctor.
- **Their bleeding is too heavy.** You should see bleeding like a period on and off for up to two weeks after the procedure. But if you are filling a maxi pad end-to-end in an hour for two straight hours or passing blood clots the size of an egg, your doctor wants to know about it.
- **They feel dizzy.** If you're having heavy bleeding and you start to feel dizzy when you're walking or even sitting up, it may be a sign that you're losing too much blood too quickly.
- **They get a fever.** Call your doctor for any temperature at or above 100.4 F.

Post-procedure care

After having a D&C, be kind to yourself. You can get a note for work or school for time to physically recover. Take it easy, though you don't need to stay at home or in bed. Don't do anything extremely physical. I tell my patients no roller coasters, no horseback riding, no helping a friend move out of an apartment. But your routine activities are fine.

Some doctors say to refrain from tub baths for a week, but this is old-school nonsense, from worry about the risk of infection. No studies have scientifically proved that this is a risk. So if a hot bath is going to make you feel better, go for it.

No vaginal intercourse is another often-stated restriction that isn't based on scientific studies. However, in this case, I feel it's better to be safe than sorry, so I tell my patients not to have intercourse in the two weeks after a procedure. That said, I'm not saying no orgasms! If being close to your partner in other ways is going to be comforting during this time, by all means do what makes you feel good.

FUTURE PREGNANCIES AFTER A D&C

Many of my patients worry that choosing a procedure to manage a miscarriage risks the health of future pregnancies. They fear that the procedure may make it harder to get pregnant again or increase the risk of another miscarriage. Thankfully, this is not the case. There is no threat to your future fertility by having a D&C. Your chances of getting pregnant again aren't any different from what they were before, and there is no increased risk of a miscarriage after a first trimester D&C.

✓ QUESTIONS TO ASK YOUR DOCTOR

Bring this list of questions to your appointment when you discuss your options for surgical treatment of your miscarriage. Take notes and check off the questions as you go.

☐ If I want a procedure, will you be the one to perform it?

_____

☐ How soon can we schedule it?

_____

☐ Where will the procedure happen?

_____

_____

☐ What are my options for anesthesia?

_____

_____

_____

☐ Are there any restrictions on what I can eat or drink before the procedure?

_____

_____

☐ If I'm having anesthesia, can I drink clear liquids the morning of the procedure?

_____

_____

☐ Do I have to have someone drive me home after the procedure? Does the person driving me home need to stay in the office/clinic/hospital the whole time I'm there?

_____

_____

☐ Can I have someone in the room with me during the procedure?

_____

_____

☐ What kind of follow-up do you recommend after the procedure?

_____

_____

_____

_____

PART 3

Special circumstances

Sometimes it may seem like all the information you see on miscarriage is directed toward people with first trimester losses. But if your loss isn't the "typical" miscarriage, it's still a miscarriage all the same.

This section gives every kind of pregnancy loss its due. I'll walk through them all: what to be ready for, what it feels like, and what to expect when it's over. In some cases, even how to know when it's over is tricky, so I'll talk about that, too.

CHAPTER 7

Second trimester miscarriage

One of my partners asked me to perform a quick ultrasound on one of her patients, Grace. Grace, a hospital employee, was concerned that her baby wasn't moving as much as she thought it should. As I squeezed the ultrasound gel on her belly, I started to tell her that it's normal at 19 weeks to feel only sporadic movement, but I stopped talking when I saw the ultrasound — and the clear absence of a heartbeat. I turned to Grace. From the tears streaming down her cheeks, I knew that she saw what I saw.

So far, this book has focused on the most common kind of miscarriage — a loss in the first trimester. Most people feel after they've crossed the 12-week mark, they should be fine — and they're not wrong to feel that way. Only 2 to 3% of pregnancies are lost in the second trimester, making it much less common than miscarriages in the first trimester.

But going from a point where you're posting ultrasound pictures on social media and telling everyone your big news to receiving a miscarriage diagnosis can be twice as heartbreaking. This chapter highlights common reasons for second trimester miscarriage, options for treatment and steps to take following this type of pregnancy loss.

CAUSES OF SECOND TRIMESTER LOSSES

The reasons why people have miscarriages later in pregnancies vary, but they generally fall into four categories. You'll read about each of them starting on the next page.

(i) MEDICINE-TO-ENGLISH TRANSLATION

These basic terms will be helpful for you to understand as you read through this chapter.

Cervix. The opening to your womb (uterus), at the inside end of your vagina, that needs to open (dilate) to allow delivery of the baby and placenta.

Cervical insufficiency. Painless dilation (opening) of the cervix. Sometimes can be treated with a procedure to stitch the cervix closed. May lead to pregnancy loss.

Dilation and evacuation (D&E). A two-step process of opening (dilating) the cervix with medication or cervical dilators and removing (evacuating) the pregnancy and placenta.

Epidural. A catheter placed in your back that bathes your spinal column in a numbing medication (anesthetic) to reduce or take away pain during labor.

Labor induction. The process of starting labor contractions with medications, to make the cervix open and deliver the baby and placenta.

Laminaria. Thin twig-like pieces of sterile dried seaweed; these are the most common form of cervical dilators. They

Abnormalities in the baby

Fetal abnormalities that are chromosomal (like trisomy 13 or 18), structural (like anencephaly) or syndromic (a constellation of problems commonly seen together) can lead to a loss.

open your cervix by swelling in size like a sponge, absorbing water, and causing your cervix to release hormones that trigger it to soften and dilate. (See photo on page 121.)

Mifepristone (Mifeprex). A medication sometimes used in the medical treatment of miscarriages. Taken as a single pill in the doctor's office. Not currently available by prescription. Often called mife for short.

Misoprostol (Cytotec). A medication almost always used in the medical treatment of miscarriages. Taken as multiple pills, it's swallowed, tucked in your cheeks (buccally) or placed in your vagina. Available by prescription, but not always immediately available at the pharmacy. Often called miso for short.

Oxytocin (Pitocin). Given in a slow drip through a thin tube placed in a vein in your arm or hand (intravenous, or IV), this medication causes your cervix to dilate and your uterus to contract, starting the labor process. Also called Pit for short.

Viability. Usually refers to the ability of a baby to survive on its own. The term *threshold of viability* is the point in the pregnancy where the baby can live outside of your body, with or without medical help.

Medical illness in the pregnant person

Serious medical illnesses can lead to a loss at this point in the pregnancy. These medical conditions include those you may know you have, like diabetes, high blood pressure and autoimmune disorders like lupus.

It also includes medical conditions you might not know about, like an underlying thyroid disease. Certain viral infections like cytomegalovirus or German measles (rubella) also can cause pregnancy loss. Sometimes pregnancy-specific conditions like preeclampsia or an infection can develop. Uterine infection is a more common reason for losses in other countries, but it can happen in the U.S., too.

Structural problems with the cervix or uterus

Previous surgery on the cervix can weaken it, making it more prone to opening or dilating before it's supposed to. This is a condition called cervical insufficiency or (I *hate* this description) cervical incompetence. Certain abnormalities of the uterus, like fibroids or unusually shaped uterine cavities, can also make a pregnancy loss more likely.

Premature labor

Your pregnancy can be compromised if labor begins months too early. This can be caused by regular contractions that dilate your cervix or by breaking your water, which is known as preterm prelabor rupture of membranes (PPROM).

It's not always possible to figure out why labor or the water breaking happens in the second trimester, but both conditions will generally lead to loss of a pregnancy if they occur before 22 weeks' gestation.

MISCARRIAGE WARNING SIGNS

Many people less at than 20 weeks of pregnancy don't have any signs at all that there's anything wrong. Their miscarriages tend to be diagnosed at the time of a prenatal visit when no heartbeat is detected, and an ultrasound confirms that the pregnancy is lost. However, sometimes there are indications of trouble.

First, spotting or period-like bleeding can be a sign that the cervix is opening without labor (cervical insufficiency). In this case, the cervix starts to open early without any contractions. If it opens enough, labor follows, leading to the delivery and loss of the baby. Sometimes bleeding in pregnancy is OK. But it can be hard to tell when things aren't OK, so call your doctor's office right away.

Another indication of a miscarriage is cramping that comes and goes very regularly and is persistent. Doctors know that belly pain happens in pregnancy for a lot of reasons — most frequently gas or constipation — but pregnancy loss in the second trimester may come from early labor. So, if you ever experience cramps at regular intervals that don't get better with acetaminophen, heat packs or a hot shower, and rest, you should call your doctor immediately.

A less common but clear sign of an impending miscarriage is a sudden gush of fluid from your vagina without any signs of bleeding. This may be a sign that your membranes have ruptured, that you've "broken your water." If fluid rushes out of you — almost like you've peed yourself, but you know you didn't urinate — see your doctor right away.

The last sign of a miscarriage is no longer feeling the baby move. Most pregnant people can feel a baby moving by the 20th week of pregnancy. If it's your second or third baby, you may feel the baby moving as early as 18 weeks. If you have felt the baby moving in your pregnancy and now realize that the baby no longer is, you should contact your doctor's office and go in for an exam.

TREATMENT OPTIONS

Depending your doctor's level of experience, the option for care by another doctor at your hospital, and whether you're having any complications like signs of infection or bleeding, your options for treatment may vary.

(?) **YOU MAY BE THINKING ...**

I don't get it — my cervix may be opening, and my water may have broken, but the baby still has a heartbeat. How is this a miscarriage?

You'll hear doctors use the term *viability* when talking about your pregnancy. This is the time in development that a baby can survive outside the womb after being born, and it varies depending on the services available at the hospital. Even with the availability of an amazing neonatal intensive care unit (NICU), babies are never considered viable before 22 weeks of pregnancy. While the baby's organs have all formed, they are too immature to keep the baby alive, even in an incubator. Between 22 and 23 weeks, survival rates aren't great, and often surviving babies have lifelong health problems because of being born so early. Viability increases dramatically beyond 23 weeks.

If you are far from this point in the pregnancy, your doctors know that there is no chance of your baby surviving after delivery, so they will consider this a pregnancy loss.

There are two ways to treat a second trimester miscarriage:

1. **Induction of labor.** This happens in a hospital, very often in a women's health unit or a labor and delivery (L&D) unit.
2. **Dilation & evacuation (D&E).** This is a surgical procedure similar to the dilation and curettage (D&C) procedure discussed in Chapter 6.

Each is very safe, but both options may not be available to all people in all circumstances. Make sure that your doctor talks about all the possibilities with you.

For most people, a history of a cesarean delivery doesn't rule out either a labor induction or a surgical procedure as options. The doctors may treat your cervix a little bit differently if it's never been dilated before, but the treatment options should be the same.

What if I've had a C-section in the past?

Even if you were told that you shouldn't labor in the future because of the type of C-section you had, it's still safe for you to have either management option for a loss.

You may have heard about having a trial of labor after cesarean (TOLAC) or trying for a vaginal birth after cesarean (VBAC) from your doctor or midwife. These terms apply to trying for a natural delivery at term. Because the baby isn't full-sized in the second trimester, an induction of labor is less risky now than it would be near your due date.

Unlike in the first trimester, expectant management is a complicated choice. With an untreated second trimester miscarriage, you face two major risks: First, if your cervix is opening too early or if your water has broken, you will likely go into labor in the next 48 hours. If you don't begin labor, you are at a very high risk of an infection in your uterus that could put you at a risk of a hysterectomy, where your uterus has to be removed, or at risk of losing your life.

And second, the biggest danger of having a miscarriage on your own this far into the pregnancy is the risk of hemorrhage, especially if the placenta doesn't pass on its own. So, your health and potentially your life would be at risk if you miscarried in an elevator, in a car or on a bus during rush-hour traffic, or some other place where it would be very difficult or downright impossible to get care.

Some people with PPROM or premature dilation of the cervix can't bear to take steps to end the pregnancy and choose to wait for the body to miscarry on its own. Even though your doctor has told you that your pregnancy is ending, it's possible for your body to hold on to the pregnancy for days or even weeks. And during this time, your risk of getting an infection in your uterus rises each day. If the doctors think that trying to wait will increase the chance of the baby being born late enough to survive, this is a risk that many people are willing to take. But if you're far from delivery, waiting only puts you at risk of a serious complication, so it isn't recommended.

While you don't have to decide how to handle your miscarriage right away, I would never advise any person to wait for a miscarriage to happen on its own. You need a labor induction or a D&E to complete the miscarriage to protect your health and your uterus for future pregnancies. You'll read about each of those procedures next.

When your doctor presents your options to you, make sure that you understand each one thoroughly. Ask as many questions as you need to so that you can make the choice that's right for you. Because you're getting so much information at these visits, you may want to have a support person with you. And if you're already in the office when you get the diagnosis and begin the discussion, ask if you can "bring" in someone by cellphone. You can put your partner, your friend or your mom on speakerphone or bring someone in via video chat to participate in the discussion.

Labor induction

All obstetricians should be comfortable with inducing labor in the second trimester. Some midwives also may be comfortable with this process, though a midwife may refer you to a doctor for more-specialized care.

Most often the labor induction happens in a labor and delivery (L&D) unit at a hospital. It may seem unfair to go through labor and deliver the baby in a hospital when you might prefer to be at home and have the miscarriage more privately like you can in the first trimester. But when a pregnancy has advanced this much, the baby and the placenta are both larger, and the risk of complications is higher. It's simply not safe for you to have this delivery at home, unattended by a health care professional. In a hospital, you'll be given your own room, and you'll receive special attention from nurses trained to help you in this situation.

Doctors use many medications to kick-start labor. Often misoprostol (Cytotec) is the medication that's used. (See Chapter 5). In the second trimester, you'll need multiple doses of miso over hours or even a day or two. You'll take miso by placing tablets in your cheek (buccally) or in your vagina, with doses given every 3 to 6 hours. If your doctor has access to mifepristone (Mifeprex; see Chapter 5), giving you a dose of mife before starting the induction can make the overall process quicker. Some doctors prefer to use oxytocin (Pitocin), which is sometimes referred to simply as Pit. This medication, given through a vein in your hand or arm (via IV), is commonly used to induce labor around your due date (at term).

Inductions can be as short as 8 to 10 hours but may take as long as a couple of days, so you won't be in the hospital much longer than that. Unlike having a baby at term, you don't need to contract for as long a period of time because your cervix doesn't need to open quite so much.

Experiencing a labor induction A labor induction at this point in the pregnancy is longer and more painful than an early miscarriage, but it's physically much easier than having a baby at term. You have access to pain medications, including an epidural, at any time. And you generally can have your partner or a support person in the room with you during the induction.

The contractions may feel relatively similar to the every-two-minutes-have-to-breathe-really-hard kind of contractions you see on TV shows and in the movies. If you've had a baby before, you'll know what those feel like. If you haven't, I would describe them as intense menstrual cramps that might take your breath away. These cramps can last up to a minute, and you'll tend to have them every few minutes over the course of several hours.

Because you're not full term, delivery of the baby happens more quickly. You seldom need more than a few pushes, and the baby may come out all at once, instead of head, then shoulders, and then body. This is especially true if you're at less than 24 weeks' gestation.

In some cases, the baby and placenta deliver at the same time, but other times the placenta comes after the baby — sometimes hours later. Also, because the baby is small, you won't need a cut in your vagina to widen the opening for delivery (episiotomy). In fact, it's exceedingly uncommon to tear at all. (Small favors.)

Just like when you're having a baby under happy circumstances, you don't have to have this pain without medication if you don't want to. For most people, the pain can be managed with medications, like morphine or Demerol, injected into an IV. Some people may prefer an epidural so that they won't feel anything. This may or may not be available to you at your hospital, but it's something that you can talk to your doctor about.

Recovery after an induction You may be able to go home within hours of giving birth. Most of the time, that's the case. Your medical team will want to make sure that your bleeding is under control, that you're not showing any signs of infection, and that, overall, you're recovering appropriately. But there's no reason that you must stay overnight in the hospital if you don't want to. Many people want to be home with their families after going through such a loss, especially if they have other children at home.

You'll want to take it easy for a few days, with no heavy lifting or heavy physical exertion for a week. That includes pelvic rest for two weeks, which means nothing in your vagina — no intercourse, no tampons or menstrual cup, and no douching — to allow the bulk of the post-pregnancy bleeding to resolve.

But you don't need to be home in bed for weeks. You'll be able to resume your usual activities, including work, within 3 to 7 days after delivery, even if you are able to take more time off to heal. It may not seem fair that your body recovers so quickly when your heart may still be hurting. If you have sick time from work or can stay out of work or school with the help of a doctor's note, take the time you need to recover emotionally, too.

Dilation and evacuation (D&E)

The alternative to labor induction is a surgical procedure to remove the pregnancy. This procedure is like the one that happens in the first trimester, but instead of being a dilation and curettage (D&C, see Chapter 6), it's a dilation and evacuation (D&E).

Unlike in the first trimester, where many doctors will give you the option of an in-office procedure, losses in the second trimester are generally treated in a surgical unit or operating room. A more advanced pregnancy and a larger placenta carry a higher risk of bleeding and requires a more technical surgery, so it's safer for you to have a higher level of care. However, the surgical prep will likely happen in your doctor's office.

Pre-procedure prep There are two ways to perform this cervical prep: with placement of cervical dilator devices or with cervical softening or ripening medications. Both allow the cervix to open so that the pregnancy can be passed much more easily and safely during the surgery the next day.

Cervical dilator placement During this procedure, performed in the office the day before your planned surgery, your doctor places dilators into your cervix to encourage your cervix to dilate naturally. A dilator is about the size of a matchstick. There's no cutting involved — the doctor just slips the dilators into the natural opening of your cervix. Often doctors place an antiseptic-soaked gauze sponge in the vagina to help keep the dilators in place before they start expanding. This procedure is performed most of the time under local anesthesia and only takes about five minutes. Every doctor's office is different, but in general, you can have your partner or a support person with you during the placement of the cervical dilators in the office.

Overnight, the dilators will soak up vaginal fluid and expand, slowly opening your cervix. During this time, you can expect cramping pain and light bleeding, but neither should be intense. Your doctor may offer you a prescription for ibuprofen or another anti-inflammatory to help with comfort. You can get these medications over the counter, but the prescription-strength dose is higher and may be more effective.

Sometimes you'll feel pressure on your rectum from the dilators, and if you feel the urge to poop, go ahead and try — you won't push the dilators out. You can shower overnight, but no tub baths, as the water might enter your vagina and cause the dilators to expand too quickly.

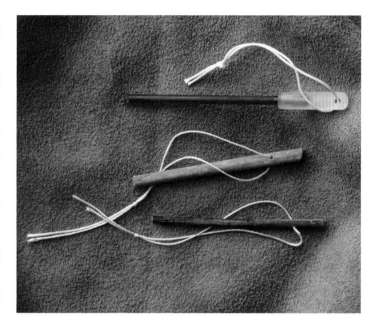
Sometimes, the gauze or the dilators start to come out before the surgery. If this happens, don't panic — it's often a sign that the dilators worked and your cervix is opening. If you feel the gauze starting to come out of your body, remove it and throw it away. If any dilators start to follow, place them in a baggie and bring them into your doctor. Your doctor knows how many dilators were placed inside you, and he or she will want to account for all of them to make sure nothing gets left behind.

If your loss happens in the first part of the second trimester, your doctor may use a fast-acting type of cervical dilator called

Dilapan. These dilate your cervix in 3 to 4 hours, which means you don't have to wait overnight. Using Dilapan will allow you to have your dilator placement and your D&E procedure in the same day.

Cervical softening medications Another option for getting your cervix ready is to take medications by mouth. Either miso or mife may be used, and both medications have a similar effect on your cervix.

If you're in the later part of the second trimester, your doctor may use both cervical dilators and softening medications to achieve maximum dilation of your cervix to accommodate the larger baby.

In addition to cervical prep, you'll need to have an empty stomach when you arrive for the surgery the next day. This usually means nothing to eat or drink after midnight the night before surgery. You'll also need to have someone with you to take you home, since you'll be sedated during the procedure. It won't be safe for you to drive, take a taxi or use public transportation afterward.

You should also prepare for a lot of waiting. Hospitals and clinics are typically not the most efficient places. It can be frustrating when on a day that you want everything to happen quickly — to get it over with — you may end up spending a lot of hours just sitting and waiting. Feel free to come armed with a book, magazine, or a smartphone or tablet full of music, TV shows and movies, and headphones to keep you occupied while you're waiting. Just be sure to download any content ahead of time. Hospitals have notoriously poor to nonexistent cellphone reception, so you can't rely on streamed content for distraction.

Experiencing a D&E In the surgical unit or the operating suite, you will have an IV placed in your hand or arm. You'll sometimes meet the anesthesia team, who will talk to you about the sedation you're going to receive. Most people undergoing a D&E will be offered sedation, either through sedative drugs in the IV or deeper sedation by an anesthesiologist. The difference between the two? Sedative drugs will make you sleepy, but you're often somewhat awake. Deep or general sedation makes it so you're not awake at all. Which option you receive depends on the type of operating room and the staff in the room with you during the procedure. Whether or not you're fully asleep, the sedation will make you more comfortable during the procedure.

After you've been given sedation, your doctor performs an exam to take out any of the overnight dilators, assess your cervix and confirm that no other dilation is needed. Then members of your care team place a speculum in your vagina and clean your cervix and vagina with soap. Next, they may inject local anesthesic around your cervix to provide a better level of pain control. Your doctor can then dilate your cervix further with dilators if a larger opening is needed to do the procedure safely. Finally, your doctor uses a combination of suction and instruments called forceps to perform the evacuation of the pregnancy.

In the first steps of the procedure, if you're somewhat awake, the most common sensation is cramping that's like menstrual cramps, but more intense. As the procedure goes on, you may feel pressure and pulling sensations, and occasional sharp pain. Let your doctor know how you're feeling, so you can get more pain medication if you need it. The worst of the pain is at the end of the procedure, after the delivery, when your uterus shrinks back down to usual size. Generally, the procedure lasts 15 to 20 minutes from start to finish.

On the procedure day itself, you may be able to have your partner or a support person be with you while you're waiting, but it's likely that no one will be allowed to be with you in the procedure room. And if you're having your procedure in a place where many other patients are waiting for procedures in the same room, the person with you will need to wait in the waiting room until your procedure is finished.

Recovery after a D&E When the procedure is over, you'll be taken to a recovery area to wake up from the anesthesia you received. Before you're sent home, your team will want to make sure that you can eat, drink and pee on your own and that you can walk without wobbling. You're going to want to recover for the rest of the day at home after this procedure.

Most of your recovery has to do with the leftover effects of anesthesia. Sedation can make you feel groggy for the rest of the day and sometimes even the next day, so don't make any plans to drive or to do anything that requires difficult thinking. It's also not uncommon to feel nauseous after surgery, so if you're feeling queasy when you're being discharged from the hospital, ask for a prescription for anti-nausea medication.

Bleeding and cramping after this procedure should generally be at the intensity of a typical period, with moderate blood flow and moderate cramps. Both signs and symptoms can last up to two weeks on and off, but by the end of that, your flow will likely be only spotting or will have stopped altogether.

Procedure risks

While both labor inductions and D&Es are safe, D&Es have slightly lower complication rates. When doctors get to control all aspects of the process, there tends to be less risk of hemorrhage or other complications, but I don't want this to deter you from having a labor induction, if that's what's important to you. Both procedures have a risk of bleeding and infection, as well as a risk of a blood transfusion, if you were to have very heavy bleeding.

The additional risk with labor induction is something called retained placenta. This scenario occurs when the baby is delivered, but the placenta gets stuck. Often, the placenta will come out, given enough time and maybe a dose of medication to help your uterus deliver the placenta. But if that doesn't work, you may need to have a D&E to remove it. Even having this "double procedure," of an induction and D&E, isn't any riskier to your health or your fertility. Needing to have two procedures is a bummer, but it doesn't hurt you.

The additional risk with a surgical procedure is called perforation, where the instruments make a small hole in the wall of the uterus. Perforation is a rare complication (less than 1 in 500 surgeries) but might require an additional surgery to confirm there are no additional injuries.

With either procedure, your doctor may include removal of your uterus (hysterectomy) on the list of risks. This may sound terrifying, but this risk is actually present *anytime* you're pregnant, and is very low with a miscarriage.

Overall, the complication rates for both labor inductions and D&Es are so low and so similar that you don't need to consider them when making your decision.

Whether you choose an induction or a D&E, breast milk leakage is a common occurrence after losses in the second trimester. The hormonal shifts after the delivery of the baby leads to milk let-down, and possibly discomfort in your breasts

Is it true my breasts may leak milk after a second trimester miscarriage?

as they swell. You can help reduce how much milk your body produces by:
- Wearing a tight-fitting bra. Sports bras are perfect.
- Refraining from any stimulation of your breasts.
- Facing away from the water in the shower.

Choosing between induction and D&E

The three factors that help my patients determine the best choice for them are pain management options, whether they're awake for the miscarriage, and whether they can see the baby afterward.

Pain Patients sometimes ask me about the differences in pain between the two options. With labor induction, you can generally get whatever pain medication you want — pills, injections into your IV, or sometimes an epidural. Only an epidural will take most to all the pain away.

With a D&E, you'll experience some pain the night before the procedure as your cervix undergoes preparation with the cervical dilators. You don't receive any pain medication this night beyond ibuprofen and sometimes codeine or oxycodone, but this pain for most people is not very intense. During the procedure, if you're receiving moderate sedation, you may be aware of pain and pressure sensations. If you're able to be fully asleep (with general anesthesia), you won't feel a thing. Pain during recovery from both procedures is similar, on the scale of a bad period.

Consciousness The second factor is whether you want to be awake when you deliver. You may have pictures in your head of what you pictured your delivery would be like, surrounded by your partner, maybe your mother — all the things that were going to bring your baby into this world in a wonderful way. For some people, the thought of going through that without a baby to take home is too devastating to contemplate. For them, a surgical procedure is the only option.

However, other people feel that if they went to sleep and woke up no longer pregnant, they would feel somehow even emptier, because the pregnancy just … disappeared. If that's how you feel, then labor induction is the best option.

Seeing the baby Typically, the biggest deciding factor is whether you want to see the baby afterward, which is often not an option with a D&E. This is a very personal decision that is up to you and your partner and your family. Some people feel that seeing the baby is a vital part of this whole process. They've carried the baby inside of them for months, and they want a chance to say hello and goodbye to a baby they very much wanted.

With a labor induction, after the delivery is over and the doctors know that you're OK — meaning your bleeding isn't heavy and nothing else needs to be done to complete the birth — the doctors can give you the baby wrapped up in a blanket to look at or hold.

(?) YOU MAY BE THINKING ...

What happens to the baby after delivery or after the procedure?

Whether you elect to see the baby or not, afterward the doctors will send the baby to the pathology department of the hospital for analysis, to look for any reasons why this miscarriage might have happened. This is also where an autopsy happens if that's something your doctor thinks would be useful and you agree. After all these tests are completed, the hospital cremates the baby. This cremation doesn't usually happen in a way that you can get ashes back, though. Some families prefer to bury the baby on their own or have the baby cremated in a way that reflects their families' traditions, so let your doctor know if this is what you want. I talk about this more in Chapter 18.

At this point in the pregnancy, babies don't look like full-term newborns do. Babies at this stage are fully formed but are very thin because they haven't yet developed the layers of fat that come in the third trimester. Often, babies look dark because of how transparent their skin is — you can see their muscles through their skin.

If you don't want to see the baby after delivery, if you feel like it will just break your heart even further, there's no reason to. Some people feel like they want to see the baby for closure, but you know what's best for you and your family. And your doctors should abide by your wishes.

If you aren't sure whether you want to see the baby, it's often possible for the staff to take photographs of your baby. This way, if you decide to not look at the baby while you're in the hospital but change your mind at a later point, you'll have the opportunity.

When it comes to a D&E, the situation is usually different. It's common for the baby to come out in separate parts, making it impossible to see the baby's face or hold the baby. You have every right to see them, but I want you to be prepared that it may not be what you expect or hope for.

If there's any chance that you think you want to hold the baby to say goodbye, ask your doctor for a labor induction. Even if you change your mind — you're not promising to see the baby at any point — it's OK to do so. Most of the time, it's not possible to see the baby whole after a D&E, so this is important to consider when you're deciding which option feels right to you.

FOLLOW-UP WITH YOUR DOCTOR

After either a labor induction or a D&E, you should schedule a follow-up visit about two weeks after the procedure. There are two reasons for this visit: First, the doctor will do an exam to be sure that you are physically healing from the pregnancy loss. Your doctor is looking to make sure your uterus has returned to its usual size, your cervix is closed, and your body is recovering the way that it should after surgery.

The second reason for a post-miscarriage visit is for your doctor to check in with you emotionally. Recovery of your heart doesn't always happen as quickly as recovery of your body. Your doctor wants to make sure that you have support for your grief and whatever emotions you're experiencing and can offer referral to support services if you need them.

Your doctor will also likely talk you through any testing results. Fair warning though: Most tests performed for miscarriage in the second trimester don't show the reasons of the loss, though it may be possible to detect a chromosome problem. Having a clear-cut answer — that we know the pregnancy wasn't typical, and that's why it was lost — may bring some comfort, but unfortunately, the reason often isn't clear.

Lastly, your doctor should talk to you about how you feel about getting pregnant again. Some people will want to get pregnant again right away. If this is how you feel, there's no reason to wait. You can get pregnant again as soon as your next cycle. But if you feel you need more time to recover before facing the idea of pregnancy again, your doctor can talk to you about birth control so that you can choose when to try again.

⊘ QUESTIONS TO ASK YOUR DOCTOR

Bring this list of questions regarding second trimester loss to your appointment. Take notes and check off the questions as you go.

☐ What kind of testing can be done to find out the reason why the baby died?

_____

_____

☐ How long will it take to get the results of the tests back?

_____

_____

If you're considering a labor induction, ask:

☐ Where would the induction take place?

_____

☐ How soon could I be admitted to the hospital?

_____

☐ Would you be the one caring for me in the hospital, or would it be someone else?

_____

_____

☐ What are my options for seeing the baby after the delivery?

_____

_____

If you're considering a D&E, ask:

☐ Where would the procedure take place?

_____

☐ How soon could it be scheduled?

_____

☐ Can you perform a D&E, or do you need to refer me to someone else?

_____

☐ What are my anesthesia options?

_____

_____

☐ Is it possible to see the baby after delivery?

_____

_____

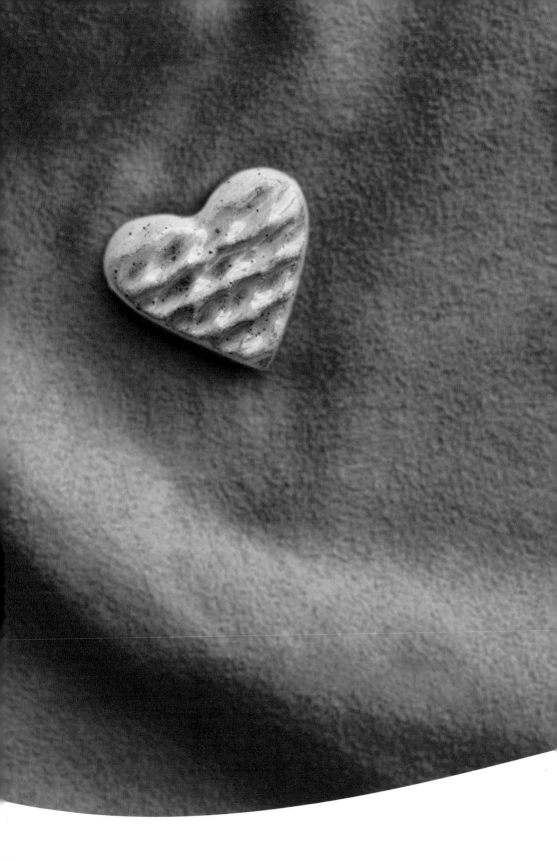

CHAPTER 8

Third trimester miscarriage

I wheeled in the ultrasound machine to examine Hannah after a nurse had trouble finding the baby's heartbeat. Hannah began talking quickly about how busy she had been over the weekend getting the house ready for the baby, whose due date was in a month. She swore she felt the baby moving as she usually did right up until this morning, but when we saw no heartbeat on the ultrasound screen, she let out a piercing cry.

For many people, making it to the third trimester of pregnancy offers a feeling of safety. You're starting to talk about delivery and maybe starting to take birthing classes. You may start thinking about having a baby shower. Even if your pregnancy developed complications at this point and you had to deliver early, the baby would probably make it. Having made it this far, you feel like you're home free. So, being told at this point in the pregnancy that you've lost the baby can be the most devastating news of all.

In the third trimester, doctors start to use the term *stillbirth* when talking about a miscarriage at this point in the pregnancy. Technically, a stillbirth is whenever a baby dies in the womb after 20 weeks of pregnancy. While most stillbirths happen before a person goes into labor, a small number of stillbirths happen during labor and birth.

Stillbirths affect about 1 in 160 pregnancies each year in the United States. That represents about 1% of all pregnancies, or 26,000 babies, annually in the U.S. alone.

STILLBIRTH RISK FACTORS

Having a risk factor doesn't mean you're destined to have a pregnancy loss, but it does increase the chances of having a

---

(i) MEDICINE-TO-ENGLISH TRANSLATION

These basic terms will be helpful for you to understand as you read through this chapter.

Cervical balloon. A small inflatable balloon at the end of a tube that can be placed through your cervix to start the process of opening (dilation).

Cervix. The opening to your womb (uterus), at the inside end of your vagina, that needs to open (dilate) to allow delivery of the baby and placenta.

Dilation and evacuation (D&E). A two-step process of opening (dilating) your cervix with medication or cervical dilators and removing (evacuating) the pregnancy and placenta.

Epidural. A catheter placed in your back that bathes your spinal column in a numbing medication (anesthetic) to reduce or take away pain during labor.

---

complication that might lead to stillbirth in a pregnancy. The factors that put you at a higher risk of stillbirth include personal and environmental risks, health problems, and issues concerning your past pregnancies and your current one.

Here's more on each risk category.

Personal risk factors include:
- Alcohol use in pregnancy
- Using nonprescription drugs during pregnancy
- Smoking tobacco or marijuana during the three months before pregnancy or during the pregnancy itself

Labor induction. The process of starting labor contractions with medications, to make the cervix open and deliver the baby and placenta.

Misoprostol (Cytotec). A medication that causes your cervix to dilate, starting the labor process. Can be swallowed (orally), or placed in your cheeks (buccally) or in your vagina.

Oxytocin (Pitocin). Given in a slow drip through an IV line, this medication causes your cervix to dilate and your uterus to contract, starting the labor process. Also called Pit for short.

Preterm prelabor rupture of membranes (PPROM). Where the "bag of water" inside your uterus that holds the baby develops a tear ("breaking your water"), allowing the amniotic fluid surrounding the baby to escape and infection to develop.

Stillbirth. When a baby dies in the womb – *in utero*, or in the uterus) – after 20 weeks of pregnancy.

- Significant secondhand smoke exposure during pregnancy
- Chronic exposure to air pollution
- Being Black, because of stress caused by racism
- Being under 20 or over 35 years old
- Having AB blood type

Medical risk factors include:
- Having high blood pressure before pregnancy
- Having diabetes before pregnancy
- Being obese

Current pregnancy risk factors include:
- Never having given birth before
- Using assisted reproductive technology
- Being pregnant with twins, triplets or other multiples
- When the baby is small for its gestational age
- Gestational diabetes

Previous pregnancy conditions (because the universe isn't fair) include:
- Preterm birth
- Preeclampsia
- Fetal growth restriction — also called intrauterine growth restriction (IUGR)
- Previous miscarriage or stillbirth

CAUSES OF STILLBIRTH

There are many causes of stillbirth in the third trimester, but they generally fall into these four categories.

Placenta problems and umbilical cord problems

The placenta and umbilical cord transfer fluid, oxygen and nutrients from the mother to the baby and transfer waste from the baby to the mother. Problems with either of these threatens to starve or suffocate the baby.

Placenta and umbilical cord problems may be caused by:
- An infection in the amniotic fluid that then infects the placenta (and the baby)
- Inflammation, which can happen when your immune system mistakenly sees the placenta as something that's invading your body
- Blood clots
- Blood vessel problems
- When the placenta separates from the wall of the uterus before birth (placental abruption)
- Umbilical cord compression, which pinches off the flow of blood and oxygen to the baby (most often caused by a knot in the umbilical cord)

Medical conditions and pregnancy complications

Health conditions and disorders linked to stillbirth include:
- Lupus
- Thyroid disorders (like an under- or overactive thyroid)
- Thrombophilias, which make blood clots more likely
- Obesity
- Being pregnant for longer than 41 weeks
- Diabetes
- High blood pressure and preeclampsia
- Preterm labor and preterm prelabor rupture of the membranes (PPROM)
- Trauma or injuries, like being in a car accident

Infections

If you get a bacterial or viral infection during pregnancy, it can infect the baby and potentially cause a pregnancy loss. These are some of the most common infections that can cause still-birth:

- Cytomegalovirus (CMV), which is common in young children and spreads through body fluids like saliva, semen, mucus, urine and blood
- Parvovirus infection (fifth disease), which spreads through the air from an infected person's cough or sneeze
- Genital infections like herpes or syphilis, which spread through sexual contact
- Urinary tract infections, often where healthy bacteria in the vagina spread to infect your bladder
- Listeriosis, which spreads through infected food products — most often deli meats and unpasteurized dairy products
- Toxoplasmosis, which you get from eating undercooked meat or not washing hands after touching cat poop

Fetal conditions

This is a common category for stillbirth that can't be predicted and often can't be detected prenatally. Some of the most common fetal conditions linked to stillbirth are:
- Birth defects and genetic conditions
- Fetal growth restriction — also called intrauterine growth restriction (IUGR) — where the baby is not growing like it should be
- When the baby doesn't get enough oxygen during labor and birth

BEING DIAGNOSED WITH A STILLBIRTH

The diagnosis of a stillbirth is painfully simple. You may notice that the baby's not moving and go into your doctor's office for a check. Or it may be at a routine visit, where the doctor can't find the heartbeat with a handheld wand that uses ultrasound waves to detect the fetal heartbeat (Doppler monitor) and sends you for an ultrasound. In either case, an ultrasound exam will show that the baby's heartbeat has stopped. Often, two people will look at the ultrasound to make sure that they get the diagnosis right, because they would never want to tell you this kind of news and be wrong.

When you get the news from your doctor, you don't have to decide in that moment how you want to manage your miscarriage. The news can be shocking, and you may need some time to process. It's perfectly fine to talk to your partner and your family about what's happening before you decide what to do next. Deciding within two weeks is usually considered safe. If you don't want to delay your decision but don't have your support person with you, ask if you can bring your support person into the discussion via speakerphone or video chat.

At this point in the pregnancy, you have fewer options than you do with a miscarriage earlier in the pregnancy. You have only two choices:

Labor induction When you talk with your doctor, the two of you together will decide when the best time is for you to go to the hospital. You may go right over after you've had an ultrasound and start the induction process right away. Many people don't feel comfortable waiting once they know that the baby has died. They just want to be admitted to the hospital and plan the delivery. But you may want to go home first and talk to your family, pack your bag, and then go to the hospital. You may even want to wait a few days, if there's something else going on in your life that you want to take care of first.

Expectant management You can wait to go into labor naturally, which will usually happen within two weeks of the diagnosis of the stillbirth. Once you go into labor, you can go to the hospital for the delivery. If you haven't gone into labor on your own after two weeks, your risk of complications increases. At that point, I would recommend labor induction.

Experiencing labor induction

If you have a choice of when to come into the hospital, I recommend coming in the evening when it's quieter. Coming in at night gives the doctors a chance to time the labor so that you deliver the following morning, though it doesn't always work out perfectly. You will usually be given a private room on the labor and delivery (L&D) unit, usually as far from the hustle and bustle as possible. You can typically have your partner and any support people by your side during this process.

Being admitted to L&D — a place you may have toured as part of childbirth classes — may feel cruel, as you will be surrounded by women who are having healthy babies. But this is the place in the hospital with the doctors and nurses who know exactly how to take care of you. They know what you're going through, and they can attend to all your physical and emotional needs, so this really is the place where you want to be.

Doctors will most often use either medications or a procedure to induce labor:
- **Oxytocin** (Pitocin or Pit), a medication given in a slow drip through a small tube that's placed in your hand or arm (IV line) that starts labor contractions.
- **Misoprostol (Cytotec).** This drug, also known as miso, causes your cervix to dilate, starting the labor process.
- **Cervical balloon,** known as a Foley balloon or a Cook catheter, causes your cervix to release hormones that begin cervical dilatation and then labor.

Which approach your doctor uses depends on how far along in the pregnancy you are, whether you're showing any signs of labor, and whether you've had one or more previous C-sections. It's unlikely that doctors will give you a choice — they're going to choose whichever one they think is safest and most effective for you. Make sure your doctor explains the medications or procedure to you, and what you may experience.

If you're earlier in the third trimester or your body is naturally preparing to give birth, a labor induction may be as short as eight hours. However, if you're later or your body isn't ready for labor, it can take as long as two days. Doctors will monitor you frequently during this time to make sure that you're not getting a fever or showing any other signs of being sick. They'll check your cervix periodically to see if you're dilating and to assess the progress of your labor. They may change the medications or increase the dosage if your labor is progressing slowly.

Overall, a labor induction for a pregnancy loss may feel like what labor feels like in healthy pregnancies, especially if you're eight or nine months pregnant. If you're earlier in the third trimester, then the process may be shorter and slightly less intense. But in either case, eventually contractions are going to

BABIES WHO DIE DURING LABOR

It's very unusual, but not impossible, for a baby to die once labor begins. Some patients will have the baby's heartbeat monitored every 15 minutes without monitoring in between. Other patients will have continuous monitoring, where the baby's heartbeat is monitored all the time. There's no scientific evidence that one method is better than another in terms of safety.

It can be hard to detect the heartbeat in some babies, either because of the mom's weight or the position of the baby. And sometimes when the doctors think they're monitoring the baby's heartbeat, they're in fact monitoring the mom's heartbeat. While it's rare, it's possible for a baby to have a complication during labor and die before the doctors notice that the heartbeat is gone.

start that will be 1 or 2 minutes apart, last about a minute, and take your breath away.

I went to labor classes to get ready to give birth, but how does it feel when the baby has died?

Any techniques you learned in your labor classes or that you used in previous deliveries are just as helpful here. Coping with the pain may involve walking around, sitting on a labor ball or having your partner rub your back. You typically don't need to stay in bed throughout the labor process, since that sometimes makes the pain worse. Some hospitals will give you the opportunity to labor in the shower or in a tub, depending on what the L&D unit looks like. You don't need to be monitored as closely when you are being induced for a stillbirth, so you won't be strapped to the bed or connected to monitors, and you may feel free to move about your room and even the hallways.

Pain management Doctors will most likely offer you a range of pain medication choices. In many situations, you can get an epidural, just as you would with a usual labor. If you choose the epidural, you won't be able to walk around, so you'll only want this option if maximum pain control is the most important thing to you. Doctors may also be able to give you IV medications to help with the pain of the contractions. These may make you sleepy, but won't make your legs numb. You'll still be able to get up to go to the bathroom and walk around.

Some people choose not to have pain medication at all. They don't want to have the experience dulled, and they always want to be aware of what's happening. This choice is completely fine as well. It's also OK to change your mind about wanting pain medication once labor begins.

Seeing or not seeing the baby Once you deliver the baby, the next big decision you'll likely make is whether you want to see

I can't believe you're telling me that I have to go through labor for a baby that I can't take home. Why can't I just have a C-section?

This is one of the hardest questions I get when I'm taking care of a patient with a stillbirth. I completely understand why the idea of putting you through labor seems cruel when you're not going to have the happy outcome that you wanted. But the C-section was developed as a technique to try to deliver the baby safely during a complicated or dangerous delivery. The C-section was never meant to be good for the mother. In fact, a C-section has serious immediate and long-term risks to the mother's health.

Once the baby is no longer alive, you are the only patient your doctor is taking care of. And your doctor should only want to do things that are the absolute safest for you. Even though it may feel like emotional torture to deliver a stillbirth, labor is by far the safest option. After all, with a C-section, your healing will take longer and will likely cause more pain and possible problems in your next pregnancy. Doctors tend to reserve C-sections for people with severe complications during an induction for a stillbirth.

the baby. This is a very personal decision that's up to you and your partner and your family. Some people feel that seeing the baby is a vital part of this whole process. This is a baby they've carried inside of them for months, and they want a chance to say hello and goodbye. In this case, after the delivery is over and the doctors know that you are OK — meaning your bleeding isn't heavy and nothing else needs to be done to complete the birth — the doctors can give you the baby wrapped up in a blanket to hold and so that you can say goodbye. Many people want to see the baby to help with closure of the pregnancy.

If you don't want to see the baby after delivery, if you feel like it will just break your heart even further, you don't have to. You know what's best for you and your family, and your doctors will abide by your wishes. The staff could also take photos of the baby for you and hold onto them in case you ever change your mind.

Afterward, the doctors will send the baby to the pathology department at the hospital. There, pathologists analyze the baby and try to determine why the stillbirth occurred. This is also where an autopsy happens if that's something you and your doctor think would be useful.

After all these tests are over, the hospital cremates the baby. This cremation doesn't generally happen in a way that you can get ashes back, though. Some families prefer to bury the baby on their own or have the baby cremated in a way that reflects their families' traditions, so let your doctor know if this is the outcome you want. I talk about this more in Chapter 18.

Recovery after an induction You may be able to go home the same day you give birth. Most of the time, that's the case. Your medical team will want to make sure that your bleeding is under control, that you're not showing any signs of infection, and that, overall, you're recovering appropriately. You don't have to stay overnight in the hospital if you don't want to. Many people want to be home with their families after going through such a loss, especially if they have other children at home.

Recovering from a stillbirth, especially in the eighth or ninth month of pregnancy, is like recovering from a delivery at term. You'll want to take it easy, with no heavy lifting or extreme physical exertion for a week. This also means pelvic rest for two weeks, which means nothing in your vagina — no intercourse, no tampons or menstrual cups, and no douching — to allow most of the post-pregnancy bleeding to resolve. Physically, you'll start feeling better by then, though it may take more time to recover emotionally. I wasn't ready to go back to work until a full eight weeks after my third trimester loss and was lucky that my employer was willing to give me the standard maternity leave.

A nasty surprise that sometimes happens after a stillbirth is that your breasts may leak milk. Your body just hasn't caught up with the loss of the baby yet. The hormonal shifts after delivery lead to milk let-down and possibly discomfort in your breasts as they swell.

You can help reduce how much milk your body produces by wearing a tight-fitting bra (a sport bra is great), refraining from any stimulation of your breasts, and facing away from the water in the shower, since heat can cause more milk let-down.

One of the emotional parts of recovery after a stillbirth is what to do with all the baby-related items you have at home. You may have only a box of diapers and some clothes, or you may have fully outfitted the nursery. I talk more about how you can think about what to do with these things in Chapter 15.

FOLLOW-UP WITH YOUR DOCTOR

Your doctor will likely screen you for postpartum depression. This is not unusual. People who have had healthy deliveries also are screened for postpartum depression to check their emotional state. Talk about your feelings with your doctor and your support network and get referrals to support services if you need them.

Your doctor will also likely perform a standard postpartum physical exam that includes a breast exam and a pelvic exam.

Your doctor is looking to make sure that your uterus has returned to its usual size, your cervix is closed and your bleeding is a typical amount. You can probably get away with not having a speculum exam if you didn't experience any tearing during the birth.

Your doctor will also likely talk to you about the results of any testing done while you were in the hospital. These may include results of your blood tests, the placental examination, and the autopsy of the baby, if one was performed. The results of genetic testing often take many weeks to return, so your doctor may follow up those results with you at a later visit.

At this visit, your doctor can refill any prescriptions you may need. Your doctor may also gently ask whether you're interested in contraception. Doctors bring this up for two reasons. First, they know that many patients aren't emotionally ready to face another pregnancy quickly. Second, it's unclear what the risks are to another pregnancy if a person gets pregnant sooner than 18 months after delivery of a stillbirth. Some studies (but not all) show that a person may be at risk of complications if pregnancy occurs before 18 months from delivery.

Your body may be able to conceive about a month after a stillbirth. So if pregnancy isn't what you want, it will be good to talk through your birth control options so that you can choose when to start trying again.

IDENTIFYING THE CAUSE OF YOUR MISCARRIAGE

There are a lot of tests that doctors can suggest to try to find out why the baby died. Doctors can often figure out the cause of the stillbirth in about two-thirds of cases — which means that in a lot of cases, we never know why the stillbirth happened. So, it's important to prepare yourself to hear results that don't shed any light on the reasons for the loss.

Talk with your doctor before your labor begins about the kinds of tests you might want to have. Tests include:

Amniocentesis

Sampling the amniotic fluid around the baby is the most accurate way to run chromosomal tests to see if there were any genetic anomalies. The fluid can be tested for infection, too. This test is often done before labor.

Genetic testing

In addition to testing the amniotic fluid, your doctor may offer you and your partner chromosome testing to see whether either of you carries an alteration in your genes that may put you at risk of stillbirth in the future.

Placental examination

The placenta can be examined after birth to look for abnormalities with the placental tissue or the umbilical cord. When an amniocentesis isn't performed before delivery, the placenta itself can be tested for infection and genetic abnormalities.

Autopsy

With this exam, the pathologist checks your baby's organs for signs of birth defects or other conditions that negatively affect how the body develops or works. Some birth defects are so severe that they cause death to the fetus or to a newborn shortly after birth. An autopsy not only helps figure out the reason for this stillbirth but also helps determine if you're at increased risk of another loss in the future.

⊘ QUESTIONS TO ASK YOUR DOCTOR

Bring this list of questions regarding management of still-birth to your appointment. Take notes and check off the questions as you go.

☐ Where will the labor induction take place?

_____

☐ How soon can I be admitted to the hospital?

_____

_____

☐ Can I wait a few days before being admitted if I want to?

_____

_____

☐ Will you be the one caring for me in the hospital, or will it be someone else?

_____

_____

☐ What medications for starting labor are the safest ones for me?

_____

☐ What are my options for pain medication? Can I get an epidural, if I want one?

_____

_____

_____

☐ Who can stay with me in the hospital during my labor?

_____

_____

☐ What are my options for seeing the baby after delivery? Can other people come see the baby?

_____

_____

_____

☐ What kind of testing can be done to find out the reason why the baby died?

_____

_____

_____

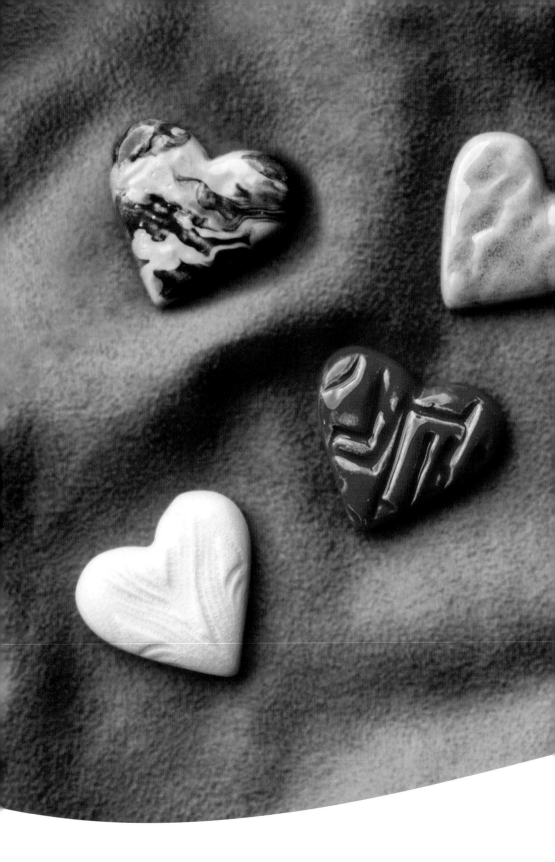

CHAPTER 9

Recurrent pregnancy loss

Imani came to me for an ultrasound because she had spotting early in her pregnancy. She had had two children with her first husband years ago and married the "true love of her life" two years prior. Since then, she had been trying to get pregnant; she had a miscarriage six months ago and was thrilled to be pregnant now. The ultrasound, however, revealed a fetus with no heartbeat. "Not again," she wept. "I can't believe it's happening again."

After a miscarriage, most people go on to have a perfectly healthy pregnancy the next time. But, if you're one of the few who is diagnosed with another miscarriage, it may lead to that sinking feeling of, "Oh, no, not again." My second miscarriage happened for reasons wholly different than my first loss — likely a chromosomal problem, compared with a maternal hemorrhage — but I couldn't believe that my body was failing me again. *Three pregnancies, one baby,* I kept repeating to myself. *How many losses do I have to survive?*

Having more than one miscarriage, generally with the same partner, is called recurrent pregnancy loss, also known as recurrent miscarriage. It's much less common than a single miscarriage. Only 5% of women will have two or more miscarriages, and 2% to 3% of women will have three or more. These numbers may reassure you if you've had a single miscarriage but may make you feel alone if you've had more than one loss.

To add insult to injury, recurrent pregnancy loss is often associated with people who've used assisted reproductive technol-

---

ⓘ **MEDICINE-TO-ENGLISH TRANSLATION**

These basic terms will be helpful for you to understand as you read through this chapter.

3D ultrasound. Like a regular ultrasound, this type uses sound waves to create a picture of your uterus. The extra "dimension" allows doctors to see if there are any abnormalities inside your uterine cavity that may be causing miscarriages.

Hysterosalpingogram. A radiology procedure used to check out your uterus and fallopian tubes. Involves placing a catheter in your cervix, injecting dye and taking X-rays of your pelvis.

Hysteroscopy. Involves placing a camera into the uterus through the vagina and cervix, and then filling the uterus with fluid. This allows doctors to remove polyps and fibroids that might be causing heavy or irregular bleeding or causing miscarriages.

Sonohysterogram. An ultrasound procedure used to check out the cavity of your uterus. Involves placing a catheter into your cervix, injecting salt water (saline) and performing an ultrasound of your uterus. Also known as saline infusion sonogram.

---

ogy (ART) to get pregnant. This may be because even the best science can't completely make up for whatever the underlying cause of infertility is. Whatever the reason, doctors know that people who use in vitro fertilization and other infertility treatments face this problem more than others.

CAUSES, TESTING AND TREATMENT

After you've had two or three miscarriages, your doctor will likely suggest that you have some testing to try to figure out what's happening. Testing helps doctors figure out a cause, so if we find something we can treat, we can increase your odds of pregnancy success in the future. Frequently, when people see a specialist for recurrent loss, both they and their partners will go together for the consultation. Doctors like the opportu-

---

(?) YOU MAY BE THINKING ...

This isn't my first miscarriage, and I don't know if I'm ever going to get to be a mother.

If you've never had a healthy baby, it's so hard to think that pregnancy is never going to work for you. And if you've had more than one miscarriage, you can feel even more despondent that you're never going to be able to keep a pregnancy.

Even after two miscarriages, though, the chances are still good that you'll have a healthy pregnancy the next time. If having a baby is incredibly important to you, give yourself time to heal, both physically and emotionally, and try again. The odds are forever in your favor — I'll show you why later in the chapter.

---

nity to talk to both members of the couple about conditions that may be happening in their situation and to talk about the testing possibilities for both partners.

Recommendations for the right testing for recurrent loss are always changing. During my career, I've seen the list of recommended tests and the order in which to do them change often. Your doctor will know the most up-to-date recommendations.

There are four categories of reasons why people have multiple pregnancy losses:
- **Anatomic abnormalities,** which are physiological problems with your uterine anatomy
- **Immune conditions,** where your immune system attacks the baby's placenta
- **Hormonal imbalances,** which can either induce an immune response or lower the hormone levels that are necessary to support your pregnancy
- **Genetic abnormalities,** which affect the baby's proper development and growth

This chapter isn't meant to be a comprehensive guide to recurrent loss. Having a solid understanding of each of these issues allows you to better understand what your doctors might be telling you and also allows you to ask much better questions to determine what you want to do, if anything. For more information, see the Resources chapter later in this book.

For now, here's an overview of the reasons for recurrent pregnancy loss, along with the options for testing and possible treatments.

Anatomic abnormalities

The first category of reasons for recurrent miscarriages is anatomic, meaning a problem with your uterine anatomy. Also called uterine abnormalities, these cause about 10% to 15% of recurrent pregnancy loss.

Uterine septum One such abnormality is having a septum in your uterus. A septum is a band of fibrous tissue that comes off the top of the uterus and protrudes into the uterine cavity. Sometimes it protrudes a little, and other times it effectively divides your uterus into two spaces. This tissue doesn't get as much blood supply as the walls of the uterus, so if a pregnancy implants on the septum, it won't receive the hormones, oxygen and nutrients that the baby needs to develop normally. If an embryo implants on the regular part of the uterine wall, having a septum may or may not adversely affect the baby, depending on the size of the septum. Having a septum doesn't mean you'll have a miscarriage, but it may be the cause if you've had multiple miscarriages.

Abnormal uterus shapes A typical uterus is the shape of a pear — rounded on the top, narrowing to the cervix below. Sometimes during development — when you were just a fetus yourself — the uterus takes on an unusual shape. These shapes can include horn (unicornuate uterus), heart (bicornuate uterus) and doubled (didelphic uterus). These abnormalities often don't cause symptoms and often aren't discovered until you have an ultrasound while pregnant. A unicornuate uterus increases the risk of ectopic pregnancy, miscarriage and preterm delivery, while a bicornuate uterus may increase the risk of second trimester loss. As with a septum, an abnormally shaped uterus doesn't doom all pregnancies but may contribute to multiple losses.

Adenomyosis Another potential cause is adenomyosis, which is the cousin of endometriosis. In both conditions, small amounts of the uterine lining grow in the wrong place. In the case of adenomyosis, these bits of lining implant in the wall (muscle) of the uterus. People with adenomyosis may have no signs or symptoms or may have severe menstrual cramps or irregular, heavy periods. These signs and symptoms are caused by extra-strong contractions of the uterus because of the implants in the uterine wall. Doctors think that for some people, the presence of these implants causes the uterus to strongly contract during pregnancy, leading to miscarriage.

Fibroids For years, it was thought that fibroids, particularly ones that are large or that protrude into your uterine cavity where an embryo might implant, could also be a cause of miscarriage. However, the latest evidence casts doubt on the connection between fibroids and pregnancy loss.

Cervical insufficiency Structural cervical weakness can be a cause of recurrent miscarriage in the second trimester. Sometimes this weakness can follow an excisional procedure, such as loop electrosurgical excision procedure (LEEP) or cone biopsy on the cervix performed for abnormal Pap tests. There are other reasons for cervical weakness, including uterine anomalies and genetic disorders like Ehlers-Danlos syndrome that affect your collagen production. Though this is increasingly rare, if your mother used the medication diethylstilbestrol (DES) when pregnant with you, and you were born with a T-shaped uterus and an irregular cervix, this can be a cause. When the cervix has a structural weakness, it dilates and thins out well before the baby is mature enough to live outside your uterus, and labor begins and can't be stopped.

Testing Testing for uterine anomalies involves looking at the inside of your uterus. A 3D ultrasound or a saline infusion sonogram (also called a sonohysterogram or sonohyst) are common tests to have first. Follow-up tests may include an MRI or a hysterosalpingogram (HSG).

You may have one or more of these tests as your doctors try to determine whether there's a problem with your uterus. People with cervical insufficiency will often have many transvaginal ultrasounds when pregnant to monitor the cervix.

Treatment Treatment can involve a surgical procedure to correct the problem, like removing a uterine septum or uterine fibroid. Surgery can be done often through your cervix under moderate or deep sedation, and it generally has a short recovery period. Certain small fibroids can be removed with a procedure in a doctor's office that has hysteroscopy available. Large uterine fibroids may require more-extensive surgery. For cervical insufficiency, your doctor may talk to you about putting a stitch in your cervix to keep it closed (cerclage), but it's unclear if these stitches reduce the risk of miscarriage.

Immune conditions

Immune conditions affect about 15% to 20% of people with recurrent loss. These disorders happen when cells in the body that fight off infections (antibodies) attack healthy tissue by mistake. While researchers are investigating several kinds of immune conditions believed to cause miscarriage, the only one that doctors can currently test for is anti-phospholipid syndrome (APS). This is a condition in which your immune system mistakenly creates antibodies that make your blood much more likely to clot. These antibodies can also cause blood clots within the placenta, starving the pregnancy of the oxygen and nutrients it needs to grow.

Testing Testing for APS involves multiple criteria. To be diagnosed with the disease, you first need to have a positive blood test — the presence of one of several antibodies in two tests at least 12 weeks apart.

Next, you need to have one of the following clinical criteria:
• Vascular thrombosis, such as getting a blood clot in your leg or having a stroke
• Pregnancy complications, including the following:
    – One or more miscarriages at or beyond the 10th week of gestation

- One or more premature births of a healthy infant before the 34th week of gestation because of an unhealthy placenta (placental insufficiency) or preeclampsia or eclampsia
- Three or more unexplained consecutive miscarriages before the 10th week of pregnancy

Treatment Treatment for APS is straightforward. You can take medication to "thin" your blood and reduce the risk of blood clots forming. During your next pregnancy, you may have to take baby aspirin daily or inject a blood thinner into your leg or belly every day.

Hormonal imbalances

Hormonal imbalances (endocrine disorders) are the reason for recurrent miscarriage about 15% to 20% of the time. There are multiple hormonal conditions that doctors associate with recurrent miscarriage.

Thyroid dysfunction This can mean either having an overactive thyroid (hyperthyroidism) or an underactive thyroid (hypothyroidism). Your thyroid is a butterfly-shaped gland that sits in the front of your neck. You can see and feel it move when you swallow. These conditions may not cause you to have any symptoms. However, if you have hypothyroidism, you may feel tired, cold and constipated. If you have hyperthyroidism, you may feel warm with a racing heartbeat. In either case, a thyroid issue can cause an immune reaction in which antibodies are produced that attack the pregnancy.

High levels of prolactin This hormone is produced in a tiny, pea-sized gland at the base of your brain called the pituitary gland. Too much prolactin can cause decreased sex drive, vaginal dryness, irregular or no periods, or even the production of breast milk when you're not pregnant. It's possible that high levels of prolactin decrease the amount of estrogen produced by your ovary, causing a miscarriage.

Polycystic ovary syndrome (PCOS) This hormonal imbalance can cause your ovaries to develop multiple cysts and not release an egg (ovulate) each cycle. People with PCOS often have irregular periods and symptoms of high levels of testosterone, including acne, hirsutism, and male-pattern hair loss. Doctors think that PCOS causes high levels of hormones that affect the lining of the uterus, making it unable to sustain a pregnancy.

Uncontrolled diabetes It's believed that the high levels of blood sugar caused by poorly controlled diabetes increase the risk of miscarriage. High blood sugar levels cause blood vessel disease (constriction), which starves the pregnancy of nutrients and oxygen, leading to miscarriage. People with diabetes that's well-controlled don't have an increased risk of miscarriage.

Testing If your doctor suspects that you have one of these illnesses based on your history and symptoms, testing for all these conditions is accomplished with blood tests.

Treatment Medication is used to restore the hormonal balances for thyroid and pituitary diseases and a treatment program for diabetes. PCOS treatment may require seeing a specialist in reproductive endocrinology.

Genetic abnormalities

Chromosomal problems are a big cause of miscarriage, so genetic problems are often the first culprit people think of when they have multiple losses.

While most chromosomal issues in an embryo are the result of a random error in development, it is possible that one or both parents have an imbalance of chromosomes that carries a higher chance of miscarriage. However, genetic problems affect only 3% to 5% of couples with recurrent miscarriage. When pregnancy loss has a genetic cause, most of the time it doesn't have anything to do with you or your partner. While there are investigations underway into a range of genetic factors that may cause recurrent miscarriage, there are two abnormalities that are the most common risk factors: balanced translocation and chromosomal inversion.

Balanced translocation The most common genetic condition linked to repeat miscarriages is called a balanced translocation. This is when one parent's chromosome swaps genetic material with another of his or her chromosomes. In this situation, you have all the information you need to be a healthy human, with no evidence of this mystery in your genetics. But a high percentage of eggs or sperm are missing a significant amount of genetic material.

A pregnancy that involves a parent with balanced translocation can end one of three ways:
1. With a genetically healthy pregnancy.
2. A pregnancy in which the embryo also has a balanced translocation. These embryos grow up to be healthy but have their own risk of miscarriages when they try to conceive in adulthood.
3. A pregnancy with an embryo that has an unbalanced translocation. These embryos are missing too much genetic material to grow, and these pregnancies end in miscarriage. Fewer than 1% of these pregnancies result in a live birth.

Chromosomal inversion Another known chromosomal risk factor for recurrent miscarriage is chromosomal inversion. This is when a segment of one of the parent's chromosomes is flipped and turned around. When one parent has an inverted chromosome, the baby may be born healthy. Or the pregnancy may lead to miscarriage, if (like an unbalanced translocation) the baby is missing important genetic information.

Testing Testing involves a chromosomal analysis of the pregnancy tissue and blood tests of the parents' chromosomes to look for balanced translocation or chromosomal inversion.

Treatment This gets complicated, because when there's a chromosomal anomaly carried by you or your partner, no medicine or surgery can fix it. This imbalance is present in every cell of your body, and science hasn't yet figured out a way to make the affected eggs or sperm healthy. However, that doesn't mean that you don't have options.

(?) YOU MAY BE THINKING ...

I had two babies with my first partner, but now I've had multiple miscarriages with this partner. What gives?

When people successfully have babies but then have recurrent miscarriages later on, they're sometimes diagnosed as having secondary infertility. This doesn't mean that they can't get pregnant, but rather that they can't seem to continue a pregnancy this time. Having had babies successfully in the past gives your doctors a lot of optimism that it's going to happen again for you. It may be just the bad luck I talked about earlier — like lightning striking multiple times — or it may point to a problem with your partner.

Undergoing a checkup for why a pregnancy might not be happening is a really hard thing for a lot of people to do. Have a long talk with your sweetie, and if having a baby together is important to both of you, encourage your partner to see a primary care doctor, a urologist or even an infertility doctor for additional testing.

Couples who receive a diagnosis of balanced translocation or chromosomal inversion either hope for the best — they simply try to get pregnant and hope that the pregnancy is healthy — or they consider undergoing in vitro fertilization (IVF). When a couple undergoes IVF, embryos can be screened for abnormalities. This process is known as preimplantation genetic diagnosis (PGD). This screening takes a single cell from the embryo and tests its chromosomes. When the healthy embryos have been identified, one or more of them are transferred into the uterus.

WHEN THE TESTING IS NEGATIVE

After all that testing, doctors are only able to find the cause of recurrent miscarriages in roughly half of the people. The other half are given the diagnosis of unexplained recurrent pregnancy loss. It can be incredibly frustrating to walk away without a diagnosis that explains the problem after all these blood tests and imaging tests.

Most often, doctors suspect that the reason for the pregnancy losses are chromosomal problems with each individual embryo that are not destined to be repeated. While we say that lightning doesn't strike twice, it's more accurate to say that it *rarely* strikes twice. Sadly, I've had patients with multiple miscarriages where each embryo is affected with a different lethal chromosomal abnormality.

Being told you have unexplained recurrent pregnancy loss can leave you feeling adrift and not sure what to do next. Consider asking for a referral to a specialized obstetrician-gynecologist (OB-GYN) — either a reproductive endocrinologist who specializes in infertility or a maternal-fetal medicine specialist who has experience with recurrent loss. Also consider an appointment with a genetic counselor, who can talk to you about the possible role of your family's medical history.

THE NEXT PREGNANCY

When thinking about another pregnancy after recurrent miscarriages, people who are diagnosed can begin treatment for these conditions. Often a healthy pregnancy can result after just a few months.

However, if your doctors haven't been able to find a cause for your miscarriages, the only thing to do is keep trying. Hearing this advice from your doctor can sound flip. It may even sound disrespectful. But if the doctors can't find a reason for your miscarriages, there really are only these three options:

1. Try again to conceive naturally.
2. Undergo in vitro fertilization with genetic screening of the embryos.
3. Stop trying and consider other ways to expand your family, like adoption or surrogacy.

This can be a big decision, and a lot of factors will go into your thinking. You may consider your age, whether you and your partner have had any other children, whether you've thought about adoption in the past, and whether your insurance covers a few tries at IVF.

Make sure you have a whole team of medical professionals with you that you trust to give you good advice and that speak to you in a way you understand. You may have a long road ahead of you, and you want to make sure that you're in the hands of people you feel comfortable with.

CHANCES OF PREGNANCY AFTER MISCARRIAGE

When I say the odds are forever in your favor, here's why:
- After one miscarriage, 80% to 85% of people will go on to have a healthy baby.
- After two miscarriages, 70% to 75% of people will go on to have a healthy baby.
- After three miscarriages, 67% to 69% of people will go on to have a healthy baby. While 67% may not sound particularly great, it's better than a coin flip.

✓ QUESTIONS TO ASK YOUR DOCTOR

Bring this list of questions about your options for recurrent pregnancy loss to your appointment.

☐ What kind of testing do you recommend for me, based on my history?

_____

☐ Will all this testing be covered by my insurance?

_____

☐ Should I delay trying to get pregnant until the testing is complete?

_____

☐ Do you think I need to see a specialist as well?

_____

☐ Should my partner undergo testing, too?

_____

☐ Do you think it would be helpful for me to talk to a genetic counselor?

_____

_____

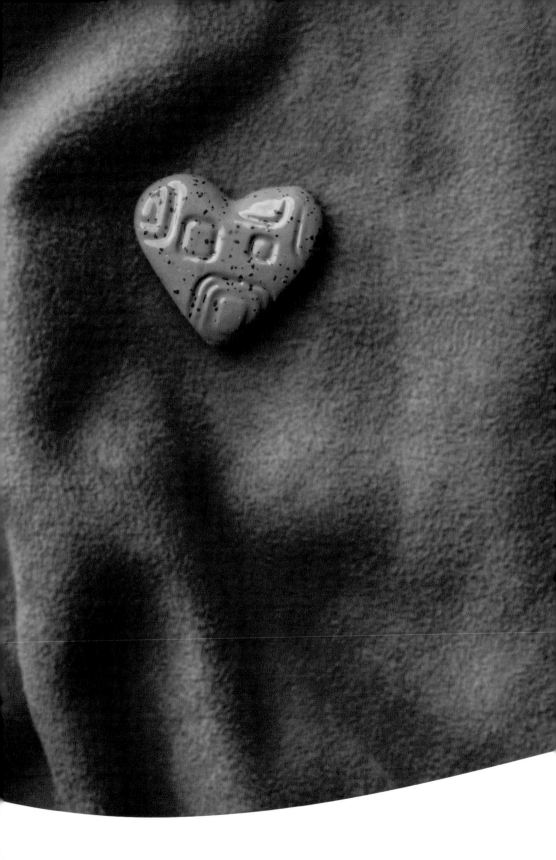

CHAPTER 10

Ectopic pregnancy

One of my nurse practitioner colleagues called me into the exam room to confirm something on her patient Jasmin's ultrasound. The nurse practitioner explained to Jasmin that she wanted a second pair of eyes on the ultrasound screen.

"But even I can see it," said Jasmin, pointing to the screen. "The pregnancy is right there!"

"Yes," I said carefully, "but that's not your uterus ... "

Earlier, I talked about using an ultrasound to discover the location of a pregnancy. That might have sounded confusing when I first brought it up. You might have asked yourself, *Where else would the pregnancy be?* Many people don't realize that a pregnancy can be somewhere other than in the uterus. And while it might sound very Ripley's Believe It or Not!, it's not as unusual as you might think.

About 2% of all pregnancies are outside the uterus. These are called ectopic pregnancies. Because they aren't in the uterus like a healthy pregnancy, ectopic pregnancies represent a much more dangerous form of a miscarriage.

Part of what makes them so threatening is that it's not unusual to have all the signs and symptoms of a typical pregnancy — nausea, breast tenderness, overwhelming fatigue. These signs and symptoms can be present regardless of whether the pregnancy is in the right spot

What does it feel like to have an ectopic? Would I still feel pregnant?

because they're related to the amount of pregnancy hormones in your blood, not the location of the pregnancy itself. You may

---

ⓘ MEDICINE-TO-ENGLISH TRANSLATION

These basic terms will be helpful for you to understand as you read through this chapter.

Ectopic pregnancy. A pregnancy growing outside of the uterine cavity.

Laparoscopy. A type of surgery that involves making a series of small (5 to 10 mm) incisions in your bellybutton and on your abdomen to perform procedures guided by a camera. Very often doesn't require an overnight hospital stay. Often referred to as "having a scope."

Methotrexate. This medication stops the growth of cells that are rapidly dividing, such as pregnancy cells. Methotrexate is given as an injection into your muscle and requires careful monitoring.

Tubal pregnancy. A pregnancy in your fallopian tube between the ovary and the uterus. The most common location of an ectopic pregnancy.

also experience mild cramping or light bleeding. But, again, you can have these signs and symptoms with a healthy pregnancy, too. So, you might not feel anything out of the ordinary until you're diagnosed with an ectopic pregnancy.

HOW ECTOPIC PREGNANCIES COME TO BE

Understanding ectopic pregnancy requires understanding pregnancies from the moment of fertilization (conception) to what is the medical start of a pregnancy (implantation). True fact: I did not learn about the details of fertilization until medical school. My Catholic school education may have been a part of it, but more likely I was too embarrassed by the whole thing during health class to pay close attention. So, if you're like me, this section is for you!

When your ovary releases an egg (ovulation), the end of the fallopian tube sweeps the egg up into the end of the tube. The egg then slowly makes its way down the length of the tube. After ejaculation, the sperm swim to the back of the vagina and through the cervix into the uterus and then into the tube to fertilize the egg. That's right — fertilization occurs *in the tube,* not in the uterus. From here, the now-fertilized egg usually continues to make its way down the tube to the uterus. Once there, it implants and the cells begin to divide, and the pregnancy (gestational) sac starts to form.

Here's where things can get complicated. Sometimes, that fertilized egg never makes it into the uterus. It stays right where it is and implants in the wall of the fallopian tube and starts to grow there. This is called a tubal pregnancy, and it's the most common type of ectopic pregnancy.

This is a serious problem because only your uterus is designed to grow a pregnancy — that's its primary purpose. (It sure isn't only to cause monthly distress for 30 years.) No other organ in your body can allow a pregnancy to grow in a healthy way. Not only is your uterus designed to protect and nurture the growing baby, but it's also designed to stretch and expand as the baby grows.

That's the chief concern with an ectopic pregnancy — left alone, the growing pregnancy will likely cause the fallopian tube it's in or the organ it's growing on to rip open (rupture), leading to life-threatening bleeding. In fact, ectopic pregnancy is one of the leading causes of death during pregnancy in the U.S. As a result, doctors take it very seriously.

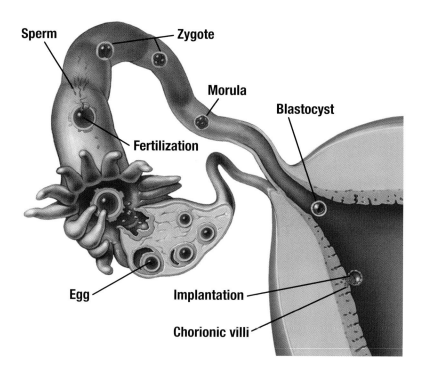

What happens during fertilization During fertilization, the sperm and egg unite in one of the fallopian tubes. Usually, the fertilized egg makes its way down the fallopian tube to the uterus. Once there, it implants and the cells begin to divide, and the pregnancy (gestational) sac starts to form.

An ectopic pregnancy is most often located in one of the fallopian tubes. But even when a fertilized egg makes it to the uterus, there can be problems. It's possible for an ectopic pregnancy to be in areas like your cervix, in the corner of your uterus near where the tube opens, in your ovaries or in the scar of a previous C-section. Ectopic pregnancies occur when the fertilized egg lands in any other place other than the healthy part of your uterus, and they're becoming increasingly common. There are even rare reports of pregnancies on other organs in your belly, including the bowel, the liver, the pancreas and the

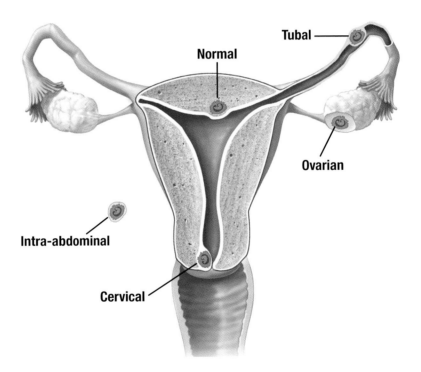

Where ectopic pregnancies can be Ectopic pregnancies are most often located in the fallopian tube, but may also be in your cervix, in the corner of your uterus, in your ovaries, or in the scar of a previous C-section. There are even rare reports of pregnancies on other organs in the belly.

spleen. These abdominal pregnancies happen when the sperm jump the gun and fertilize the egg before it's even entered the tube. The fertilized egg then bounces around in your belly and eventually lands on another organ and implants there.

ECTOPIC PREGNANCY RISK FACTORS

Having a risk factor doesn't mean you're destined to have an ectopic pregnancy, but it does increase your chances of having one.

Risk factors include:
- Having damage to your fallopian tubes, which makes it harder for the fertilized egg to make its way into your uterus without getting stuck. Tubal damage can come from:
  - Endometriosis
  - Pelvic inflammatory disease (PID)
  - Previous surgery on your fallopian tubes, including any kind of tubal ligation or sterilization procedure, or a reversal of one
- Being over 35 years of age.
- Smoking tobacco.
- Being of nonwhite race.
- Having had an ectopic pregnancy in the past. This is the biggest risk factor of all, because whatever factor led you to have one ectopic pregnancy will still be there and put you at high risk of having another one.

CAUSES OF ECTOPICS

Why did this happen to me? Why did my pregnancy not implant where it was supposed to?

More so than other miscarriages, doctors aren't sure why ectopic pregnancies occur. Doctors aren't sure why the fertilized egg would choose the tube, a scar or your cervix to land on, when there's so much prime real estate in your uterus. But just as with other miscarriages, there is nothing that you did to make this pregnancy end up not healthy, or in this case, in the wrong place. Most of the risk factors for ectopic pregnancies are not things that you can change (see "Ectopic pregnancy risk factors" on the previous page).

You can't change your race, your age or your medical history. In the same way that you didn't cause this pregnancy to be ectopic in the first place, you also can't prevent other pregnancies from being ectopic. It's a good idea to eat well, sleep well, work out and lead a happy, stress-free life — would that we all lead such a life! — but these things do not protect against ectopic pregnancies, or miscarriages in general. You should not blame yourself one bit.

DIAGNOSIS

Doctors don't know for certain where a pregnancy is located until they see it on ultrasound. And if you're feeling good early in your pregnancy, you don't tend to get your first ultrasound until late in the first trimester, somewhere between 11 and 13 weeks. My patients sometimes ask me why they can't get an ultrasound as soon as they find out they're pregnant. As I mentioned early on in this book, I tell patients that I delay the first ultrasound until the end of the first trimester because we're not likely to learn anything about the health of the baby before then. A bonus is that I can perform other testing at the same time as the ultrasound — testing that gives you information about whether your pregnancy is at risk of birth defects. Most people, in other words, don't have an ultrasound until this point as long as they're feeling well.

But people who are having vaginal spotting or pelvic pain early in pregnancy often get an ultrasound, and that's because spotting and cramping are two of the signs and symptoms that

ECTOPICS ARE MISCARRIAGES, TOO

Because ectopic pregnancies are medically complicated and can become dangerous, doctors tend to spend all their time with you talking about the treatment plan. Of course, arranging for treatment is important to keep you healthy and safe. But what sometimes gets lost in the discussion of procedures and tests is that a pregnancy is being lost. While it's important to expertly treat an abnormal pregnancy, it's also important to treat the situation of the loss.

Just because an ectopic pregnancy is treated differently, medically, from a miscarriage of an inside-the-uterus pregnancy doesn't mean that you don't feel the same heartache. If you've experienced an ectopic pregnancy, know that it's absolutely OK to grieve the same way you would a typical miscarriage.

a pregnancy may be ectopic. To be clear: Cramping and spotting happen all the time in healthy pregnancies, too, so if they happen to you, don't panic. But you should see your doctor, just to be sure that the pregnancy is progressing well.

With an ectopic pregnancy, the technician may see one of two things with the ultrasound. The first possibility is nothing, which may be surprising. The uterus may look empty, and the rest of the tissues in your pelvis may look fine. In this situation, a blood test looking for pregnancy hormones can let your doctor know how far along your pregnancy has progressed, and whether he or she should be able to see a pregnancy by now. Until a pregnancy can be seen on an ultrasound, you have a *pregnancy of unknown location*. This means the pregnancy is in there somewhere, but the exact place is unclear. It's a tempo-

Why can't you just move the pregnancy into the uterus? I really want this pregnancy.

Once a pregnancy implants outside the uterus, there's no moving it. The placenta isn't attached like a sticky note that can be lifted up and moved somewhere else. The pregnancy embeds itself into the tissue in such a manner that there's no way to pull it out — even using the most advanced, careful, surgical techniques — to implant it somewhere else. Once an ectopic pregnancy is diagnosed, it should be thought of in your mind and in your heart as the same as any other miscarriage — an irreversible loss.

rary state — your pregnancy is *somewhere*, after all — and only time (and blood tests and ultrasounds) will tell if the pregnancy is in the uterus or somewhere else. The second possibility is that the technician sees the ectopic pregnancy. In this situation, the technician can see the pregnancy sac — with or without an embryo — outside of your uterus. If the technician can clearly see the ectopic pregnancy and you get your diagnosis right away, you can move to the treatment phase more quickly. But if the doctor isn't sure where the pregnancy is, you may need more blood tests and ultrasounds before your doctor knows if your pregnancy is healthy or not.

TREATMENT OPTIONS

For ectopic pregnancies, you can usually choose between taking a medication or having surgery. If you've been reading this book straight through, you know that those two choices are options for most kinds of miscarriages.

However, just like with second trimester miscarriages, watchful waiting is not an option for ectopics. It's true that there's a very slim chance that the pregnancy will resolve on its own; the tube can expel the pregnancy into the abdomen, where it's then absorbed by the body. But by far, the most common way an untreated ectopic pregnancy ends is when it ruptures your fallopian tube. Ectopics pose such a serious risk to your health and life that you can't wait it out.

Once an ectopic pregnancy is diagnosed, you must be treated in one way or another. You may have a choice between taking a medication or having surgery. But you might not be a candidate for one of the treatments for reasons related to your pregnancy or your medical history.

The treatment for ectopic pregnancy is more complex than that of a typical miscarriage, so you'll need the higher level of care a doctor provides. Make sure that you understand your options for treatment. Both choices for management are more complicated than for a miscarriage of a pregnancy in your uterus, so it's completely OK to want to ask a lot of questions.

Because you're getting so much information at this visit, you may want to bring a support person with you. You could bring your partner, your friend or your mom — anyone who can help you "get" what the doctor is saying. And if you're already having the discussion, and no one came with you to your doctor's office this day, ask if you can bring your support person into the conversation by speakerphone or video chat.

Medical treatment

Right now, there is only one medication used to treat ectopic pregnancies: methotrexate. This medication stops the growth of cells that are rapidly dividing, such as pregnancy cells. It was originally developed as a cancer drug because cancer is also a condition in which cells rapidly divide. Because of this, methotrexate is only administered in hospitals and under careful monitoring.

Methotrexate is given as an intramuscular injection, most often into your buttocks. There are a few different dosing regimens — a single injection, two doses three days apart, or multiple doses every other day for at least a week. Which schedule of treatment your doctor chooses is based in part on how far along you are in the pregnancy, your pregnancy hormone levels and the size of the sac. But in general, the further along you are, the more doses of methotrexate you usually receive.

Methotrexate works as well as surgery for ectopic pregnancies if:
- You have low pregnancy hormone levels — less than 5,000 milli-international units per milliliter (mIU/mL)
- An embryo isn't seen in the pregnancy sac, or the embryo doesn't have a heartbeat yet
- The ectopic pregnancy is small or the exact location can't be seen on an ultrasound

But if your hormone levels are high, the embryo has a heartbeat, or the pregnancy sac is large, methotrexate has a higher chance of failing. It's important to have a long conversation with your doctor about what the chances are of it working for you.

After you get your first dose of methotrexate, your doctor gives you a detailed schedule of when to come back for blood tests so that they can monitor your pregnancy hormone levels. Even though your pregnancy hormones may go up initially after you get the methotrexate, they should start to come down shortly thereafter.

When my patients learn that methotrexate is a cancer drug, many of them become concerned about its side effects. The dose used for an ectopic pregnancy isn't as high as when treating cancer. Hence, the side effects most people experience are much less intense. The most common side effect is some cramping belly pain, and this usually occurs during the first day or two of treatment. You may also start or continue to see vaginal bleeding or spotting, or have other gastrointestinal side effects, like nausea, vomiting or indigestion.

Rare side effects of methotrexate People who receive methotrexate to treat ectopic pregnancies rarely experience the more-serious side effects of the drug, but there is a small chance of experiencing the following:
• Skin sensitivity to sunlight
• Inflammation of the membrane covering the eye, which causes blurred vision
• Sore mouth and throat
• Temporary hair loss (This may be the scariest potential side effect but know that it's very rare.)
• Severe low blood counts (bone marrow suppression), which you may not know about until your next blood test
• Inflammation of the lung (pneumonitis), which may look like pneumonia

If you are experiencing any of these effects, tell your doctor.

During the methotrexate treatment period for an ectopic pregnancy, you need to avoid taking certain things to avoid harmful interactions. It's important to avoid:
• Vitamins with folic acid including all prenatal vitamins
• Alcohol
• Penicillin
• Anti-inflammatory medications like ibuprofen or naproxen

If you need pain medication for cramping during this time, acetaminophen (Tylenol) is your safest choice.

Warning signs to watch for The most important symptoms to look out for are an increase in pain in your pelvis and dizziness. These could be warning signs that the pregnancy has ruptured and you're starting to bleed internally, so it's important to call your doctor right away if you experience these symptoms.

Call your doctor after methotrexate treatment if you experience any of the following symptoms, as well. These are signs that your ectopic pregnancy is beginning to rupture, or that you're having serious side effects from the medication:

- Increased pain in your pelvis or belly that doesn't improve with a pain reliever or a hot bath
- Pain in either shoulder
- Sores in your mouth or on your lips
- Signs of unusual bleeding or bruising
- Blood in your vomit
- Blood in your urine
- Blood in your stools, or black and tarry stools

When it's over When you're taking methotrexate and having regular blood tests, your doctor will be watching the pregnancy levels between day four of treatment (with the injection day considered Day One) and day seven. Your doctor is expecting to see a 15% drop in the level of pregnancy hormone between these two tests. If your hormone levels have dropped that much in this first week, then you'll usually get blood tests on a weekly basis until the hormone level reaches essentially zero. This can take anywhere from four weeks to three months, depending on how long it takes for the pregnancy to resolve.

If your hormone levels stay steady or increase, it's a sign that the medication isn't working. You may get another dose of methotrexate, but there's a higher chance you'll need surgery.

It may be strange to rely on blood tests, rather than your symptoms, to tell you that the pregnancy is over. When you take

What if I can't come back on one of the days of the blood tests? Is that bad?

Your doctor may seem obsessive, telling you which days you must come back for testing. But there is something special about the specific values on day 4 and day 7. When doctors can see a 15% drop in the HCG levels between these two days, they know that the medication is working.

If you miss one of these blood draws, your doctor needs to guess what the levels might have been (even doctors who are supersmart aren't wizards), which makes it very hard to know if the ectopic pregnancy is being adequately treated or if you're still at risk.

If you think coming back for blood tests on a strict schedule won't work for your job, school or child care, consider choosing surgical treatment.

medication for other kinds of miscarriages, you will start to have cramping and bleeding. These changes will mark the passage of the pregnancy tissue and give you reassurance that the pregnancy is ending.

With an ectopic, though, the pregnancy doesn't pass out of your uterus, cervix and vagina as large amounts of tissue. Instead, it starts to shrink up (necrose) and eventually either passes out undetected with a period or may even be absorbed by your body. Therefore, you won't see as much bleeding or have as much pain as you would with a typical miscarriage.

However, because your uterus has prepared for a pregnancy, you will still experience some bleeding as the lining sheds, around the level of a period. The bleeding may start soon after you get your first dose of methotrexate, or it may take a few days to begin. But that isn't enough of a sign by itself to know that the medication is working. Instead, the only thing that tells your doctor that things are going in the right direction is your level of pregnancy hormones.

It can be really annoying to need so many blood tests, especially if you are working, are in school, or have kids to take care of. But those follow-up blood tests are vitally important so that you and your doctor both know that the pregnancy is resolving. One of the reasons that a person might not choose medication and may choose surgery is the difficulty of sticking to such a strict schedule. Think about this carefully as you're making this decision as to which kind of treatment you want.

Surgical treatment

Some people prefer surgery because it's a definitive treatment that they know is going to take care of the ectopic pregnancy, without multiple visits, blood tests and monitoring. If your doctor suspects that your fallopian tube has started to rupture, this is your only option.

These surgical procedures are performed in an operating room under general anesthesia, the kind where you're fully asleep. Most of the time, doctors approach surgery for an ectopic pregnancy through laparoscopy — where tiny incisions are made on your belly and long, skinny instruments are placed inside you. One of the instruments is attached to a camera so that doctors can operate by looking at a television screen. This kind of surgery is called minimally invasive, since you don't need a big incision on your belly. (Though many people reasonably consider *any* surgery to be plenty invasive.)

During surgery, if the pregnancy is in the fallopian tube, the doctor will decide between one of two procedures. The first is removal of the whole tube containing the pregnancy (salpingectomy). With this procedure, you don't risk another tubal pregnancy on that side. However, it also means that it may be harder to get pregnant in the future since your ovaries take turns ovulating and the eggs from one of your ovaries won't have a tube to easily go down to get to the uterus. I had a patient who had one tube on the left side (she had the right one removed for an ectopic pregnancy) and one ovary on the right side (because her left ovary was removed for a large cyst). She was told she wouldn't be able to get pregnant — and yet she did. So never count your eggs out — they'll try to find a way!

The other option is to make a cut into the fallopian tube and take the pregnancy out, leaving the rest of the tube behind. You might think this is the option you would want — because who wants to lose an organ that they don't need to? But there are two challenges with this approach: First, you want to be sure that the whole pregnancy is removed at the time of surgery. If your doctor leaves the tube behind, you may need to get multiple blood pregnancy tests to make sure that the pregnancy is really over. And second, because the tube is scarred from having a pregnancy in it and surgery on it, you're now at higher risk of another ectopic pregnancy in that tube going forward.

Based on research, it's not clear if taking the whole tube out or just removing the pregnancy from the tube is better for future pregnancies. Ask your doctor about the preferred approach.

Emergency surgery What I've described so far in this chapter is the typical approach. You get the diagnosis, you're stable, and you've decided to have surgery. It's likely that you'll have the surgery that day or the day after because of the immediate threat to your life that an ectopic pregnancy represents. You may be admitted to the hospital first or be taken right to the operating room and admitted to the hospital after the surgery.

Sometimes, the ectopic pregnancy isn't discovered until it has started to rupture. If this happens to you, you may feel a lot of pain and possibly be dizzy. An ultrasound will show that you're bleeding internally, and you'll need emergency surgery. It can be harder to have these conversations when the doctor is saying, "You need to have surgery *right now*," but try to get answers to your questions as best as you can. Even if your surgery is an emergency, most doctors will still use the laparoscopic approach with the small incisions. But if your doctor is worried that you're very sick and losing a lot of blood, you may have an incision like a C-section on your belly to get to the tube faster to stop the bleeding.

When it's over After your surgery, if you have had a laparoscopic procedure, you may wake up with three or four small or clear bandages covering your incisions. Some doctors use a special kind of glue to close the incisions, so you might not have any bandages.

While you may not look like you've had a big surgery, you may feel as if you did. Depending on the time of day of the procedure, you may be able to go home after you recover from the surgery and not have to be admitted at all. It's better to be in your own bed if you can be — you'll get much better rest.

Your doctor may want you to spend the night in the hospital if the procedure finished late in the day, or if the surgery took a long time or was complicated. If you lost a lot of blood during the surgery, your doctor will likely want you to stay overnight in the hospital for a blood transfusion or just to be observed more closely. Either way, if you have a laparoscopic procedure, it's unusual to stay in the hospital more than a day or two.

If you had emergency surgery, where your doctor needed to make the bigger C-section-style incision on your belly, you may have more pain. In situations like this, it's not uncommon to stay in the hospital for two or three days.

Your doctor won't want to send you home from the hospital until he or she know that you're going to be able to take care of yourself. That means you need to be able to do the following:

- You can walk around without assistance.
- You're peeing normally.
- Your appetite is returning at least somewhat (not that you have any appetite for hospital food).
- Your pain is controlled with the medications you're given.
- Your bowel function is starting to come back, which means that you can pass gas before you'll be allowed to leave the hospital, even if you don't need to poop.

Once you leave the hospital, you'll be out of work or school for two weeks or more after this procedure, depending on how you feel. Pain is common in this postoperative period, so I always recommend to my patients that they stay on top of their pain medications and take them on a regular schedule so that the pain doesn't build up and become too much to bear. Ask your doctor about pain medication before you go home.

While at home recovering, you don't need to stay in bed the whole time. In fact, bed rest is the worst thing you can do after surgery. Get up and move around. Cook if you enjoy it. Go to a movie. Watch your kids at the park, and push them on the swings.

However, you'll want to refrain from any strenuous physical activity for six weeks after surgery. This means no lifting of heavy loads of laundry or boxes, no fun outdoor activities like riding horses or roller coasters, and no strenuous physical workouts. The incisions in your skin need to close and heal completely before you start exerting any tension in your belly, otherwise you're at risk of developing a hernia. That's when abdominal tissue bulges up through the incision, like a soft lump in your belly. Your doctor can give you a note for work to help restrict your activity if you have a job that involves a serious physical component.

Your doctor will talk to you about the care of the incisions. The small incisions may need dressing changes, which isn't much different from changing an adhesive bandage, every day for up to a week. You may need to come back to the hospital to get stitches removed, depending on how your incisions were closed. The nurses should give you clear instructions before you leave the hospital on how to take care of your skin. If you don't have clear instructions or if you have any questions, call your doctor's office and ask.

Other than the restrictions you've read about, there aren't a lot of other restrictions on your activity. You won't want to get the bandages soaking wet, but you should be able to take showers. If you have bleeding that's like a period, you should be able to use tampons instead of pads if you want to. And you should be able to have sex as soon as you feel emotionally and physically ready for it. I tell my patients to wait two weeks for the incisions to heal.

TRYING AGAIN AFTER AN ECTOPIC PREGNANCY

If you've been treated with surgery for a tubal ectopic pregnancy, there's no need to wait to try for pregnancy. If you are physically and emotionally up for getting pregnant again, go for it with your next cycle.

However, my advice is different for the rare ectopic pregnancies like ones that happen in a C-section scar, inside your cervix, or in the horn of your uterus (a cornual pregnancy or an interstitial pregnancy). In those cases, your uterus has to heal. If you have any kind of ectopic pregnancy that involves trauma or damage to the uterus, I recommend waiting at least three months, if not six months, before trying to get pregnant again.

Similarly, if you've been treated with methotrexate, the standard advice is to wait at least 3 to 6 months before you try to conceive again. It's unclear if there can be residual methotrexate during these months. If a new pregnancy is exposed to methotrexate, that alone could cause a miscarriage.

As I mentioned at the start of this chapter, once you've had one ectopic pregnancy, your risk of having another one is higher. The risk of a recurrence, or a repeat of an ectopic pregnancy, is approximately 10% after having one — and increases to at least 25% after two or more previous ectopic pregnancies. These increased risks do not mean that you shouldn't try to get pregnant again, though.

✓ QUESTIONS TO ASK YOUR DOCTOR

Bring this list of questions about your options for ectopic pregnancy to your appointment. Take notes and check off the questions as you go.

☐ Do you think that methotrexate has a good chance of working for me?

_____

☐ If I choose the methotrexate option, what days do I need to return for the blood tests?

_____

☐ Do you think that one dose or two doses of methotrexate is better for me? How does that affect when I come back for more blood tests?

_____

Most of the time, your next pregnancy will be in the uterus, with no drama. It's just a note of caution that it may be prudent to have your first ultrasound sooner rather than later in your next pregnancy, to confirm that it's in the correct location.

☐ If I choose surgery, would you plan to take out just the portion of the tube where the pregnancy is implanted or the entire tube? Why?

_____

_____

_____

☐ Do you think that surgery is a safe option for me, given my medical history?

_____

☐ Would you be the one to perform the surgery, or would it be someone else?

_____

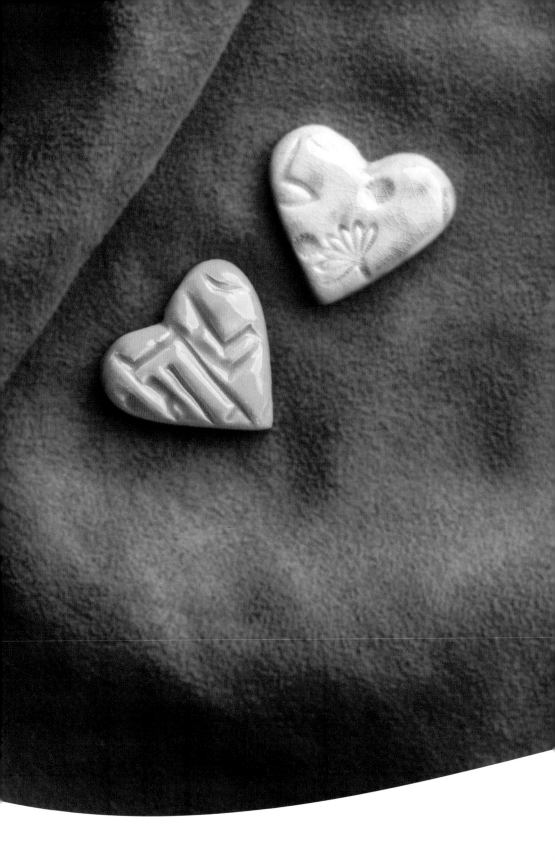

CHAPTER 11

Molar pregnancy

Lucy, age 42, was having her long-awaited first pregnancy and came to me for an ultrasound after reporting spotting to her regular OB-GYN. During the ultrasound, we both saw her uterus on the screen — no pregnancy sac was visible, and instead, the uterus had the appearance of static on a black-and-white television. "I don't understand," Lucy said anxiously. "I'm supposed to be almost three months — where's the baby?"

A molar pregnancy is a rare kind of miscarriage — only about 1 in every 1,000 pregnancies — and may be the most confusing miscarriage of all. There are some implications to your health beyond the pregnancy itself, so it's important that your doctor really gives you a good understanding of what's happening. Of course, that's what I'm here for, too.

To properly explain a molar pregnancy requires a lesson about human genetics … and possibly more than you ever wanted to know about chromosomes. In a typical pregnancy, the embryo has 23 pairs of chromosomes — the genetic ingredients for developing everything in a human body. Half of each pair comes from the mother and the other half from the father. But in a molar pregnancy, two kinds of fertilization errors can happen.

ⓘ MEDICINE-TO-ENGLISH TRANSLATION

These basic terms will be helpful for you to understand as you read through this chapter.

BHCG level. The level of the pregnancy hormone in your blood. Formal name is *beta-human chorionic gonadotropin*. Very high levels may indicate a molar pregnancy.

Choriocarcinoma. Abnormal growth of the placenta that can continue to grow even after a procedure to remove it and can become cancerous by spreading to other organs. Most often happens after a complete molar pregnancy.

Complete molar pregnancy. A pregnancy that contains only placental tissue, and no embryo or fetus. Can lead to pregnancy tissue spreading throughout the body.

Dilation and curettage (D&C). A two-step procedure of stretching open the natural opening of your cervix with dilators and then removing the pregnancy, typically with suction rather than scraping with a metal instrument (curetting). Also called vacuum or suction aspiration.

Invasive mole. Molar tissue penetrates deep into the middle layer of the uterine wall and causes heavy vaginal bleeding.

Partial molar pregnancy. A pregnancy with too many chromosomes, which can't lead to the growth of a healthy baby. An embryo or fetus may be present but won't live to be born. Also called incomplete mole.

Persistent gestational trophoblastic neoplasia. Any molar tissue that remains and continues to grow after a dilation and curettage (D&C).

In a **complete molar pregnancy,** an empty egg, where the female's chromosomes are lost or turned off, is fertilized by two sperm or just one sperm where the genetic material is duplicated. So, all the embryo's genetic material comes from the male. With this pregnancy, the placenta grows to fill the uterus. It swells and forms fluid-filled cysts — but no embryo ever grows.

In an **incomplete or partial molar pregnancy,** the egg has all the usual female chromosomes, but the sperm provides two sets of chromosomes. Most often, this happens when two sperm fertilize the egg. (Insert your own joke here about men and threesomes.) As a result, the embryo has 69 chromosomes — *way* too many for a healthy pregnancy.

RISK FACTORS FOR A MOLAR PREGNANCY

Just as with the rest of the miscarriages in this book, you did nothing to cause this to happen. You didn't choose the wrong partner. You didn't get pregnant at the wrong time. You didn't do anything during the pregnancy that made this happen.

At its core, a molar pregnancy is like other miscarriages — there's a problem with the development of the pregnancy, right from the beginning, that makes the pregnancy unhealthy. There's nothing that you can do to cause it, and there's nothing that you can do to stop it from happening, either.

People at "extreme ages," younger than age 20 or older than age 35, have a higher risk of a molar pregnancy. I put "extreme ages" in quotes because it's fairly common for people to have a baby outside of that window — I had both of my biological kids after age 35; it's normal! — but that's how doctors refer to it. People of Mexican, Southeast Asian and Filipino heritage also are more at risk of a molar pregnancy, which doctors think is because of genetic reasons.

WARNING SIGNS OF A MOLAR PREGNANCY

As with other kinds of miscarriages, you may experience vaginal bleeding or spotting, or more nausea and vomiting than you would expect from a typical pregnancy. When your doctor does a pelvic exam at your first prenatal visit, your uterus may feel larger than expected. A rapidly growing uterus may mean that you have twins, but it also may signify a molar pregnancy. On your exam, your doctor may also find that your heart rate or blood pressure is higher than usual.

If you have any of these signs and symptoms of a molar pregnancy while pregnant, call your doctor:
- Vaginal bleeding that can be bright red to dark brown
- Pelvic pressure or pain
- Severe nausea and vomiting
- Vaginal passage of grapelike cysts, although this is rare

DIAGNOSIS

A molar pregnancy is often diagnosed in the later part of the first trimester or the early part of the second trimester during an ultrasound. Sometimes the ultrasound picture is described as a snowstorm because it looks like a blizzard or TV static.

With a complete molar pregnancy, you aren't *really* pregnant — certainly not in the way you're used to thinking about pregnancy. While your body produces pregnancy hormones and tissue in your uterus, there is no baby in there and one won't ever develop. Instead, the uterus is full of placental tissue.

Partial molar pregnancies exist in a strange gray area between a healthy pregnancy and a complete molar pregnancy. Your body may produce some normal placental tissue alongside the abnormal tissue. An embryo may be developing in the uterus, but its heartbeat usually stops early in the pregnancy.

Often, a partial molar pregnancy looks the same on an ultrasound as other miscarriages do — with a gestational sac and an embryo — and it's not until after the pregnancy is removed and tested for abnormalities that you receive a diagnosis. Less often, the placenta looks unusually large and the embryo looks smaller than it should be, so your doctor might suspect a partial molar pregnancy even before the pregnancy is removed.

TREATMENT OPTIONS

Treating a molar pregnancy safely requires a surgical procedure to remove the tissue. Doctors recommend a procedure because the presence of more pregnancy tissue than in a regular miscarriage puts you at high risk of very, very heavy bleeding as your body expels the tissue.

Typically, the treatment takes place in an ambulatory surgical unit or operating room. Medications are given to you through a small, thin tube inserted into your hand or arm (IV) to stop any excessive bleeding. A procedure called dilation and curettage (D&C) removes the pregnancy with an electric suction machine. See Chapter 6 for a full description of the procedure.

Even though there isn't a choice to make about how to treat a molar pregnancy, you may want a support person with you when you're discussing it with your doctor. Bring your partner, friend, mom — anyone who can help you understand what the doctor is saying. And if you're getting the news and you're alone in the office, ask if you can bring your support person into the conversation over speakerphone or video chat.

FOLLOW-UP WITH YOUR DOCTOR

With a molar pregnancy, your doctor will monitor your pregnancy hormone levels for weeks and sometimes months. That's because in molar pregnancies, human chorionic gonadotropin (HCG) hormone levels greatly exceed those of a healthy pregnancy. They're 2 to 3 times higher, and sometimes even higher than that, compared with a healthy pregnancy.

The way the doctors know whether all the placental tissue has left your body and that nothing is sneakily growing somewhere is to follow the drop in your pregnancy hormone levels week after week after week until the level reaches zero. (Weird laboratory fact: In some hospitals, a level of less than 2 or less than 5 is interpreted the same as zero. So, your doctor may respond to a level of 3 as zero, and that's just fine.)

After your levels reach zero, you'll still have your blood checked once a month for up to six months, and sometimes a year, to be completely sure no placental tissue remains. This

---

(?) YOU MAY BE THINKING ...

Why can't I just take medication to complete the miscarriage? I don't want a procedure.

When a patient is at risk of complications, doctors want to control the circumstances as much as possible. Because the risk of heavy bleeding is so high with a molar pregnancy, the safest way to treat your miscarriage is under the direct watch of your doctor. If bleeding becomes heavy, your doctor can immediately respond by giving medications or other procedures to reduce how much blood you lose. And in the most severe cases when you've lost a lot of blood, you can get a blood transfusion. Doctors can't do any of these things if you're bleeding at home after taking medication.

---

follow-up can feel endless, but doctors need to be sure that no placental tissue remains or has spread to any other part of your body. You'll learn why this is important next.

POTENTIAL COMPLICATIONS

Besides the risk of heavy bleeding during the procedure, molar tissue could stay in the uterus and grow. This continued growth is called persistent gestational trophoblastic neoplasia (GTN). This happens in about 15% to 20% of complete molar pregnancies, and in up to 5% of partial molar pregnancies. Doctors diagnose persistent GTN by using blood tests to monitor pregnancy hormone levels. If hormone levels don't drop, or they increase, after the procedure, you may have persistent GTN.

There are two main types of persistent GTN. The most common type is an *invasive mole*. The risk of developing an invasive mole increases for people over 40, for those with a history of gestational trophoblastic disease, or for someone who is more than four months pregnant when treated. Pregnancy tissue that penetrates deep into your uterus, instead of staying on the inner lining, can cause continuous or heavy bleeding after the procedure, which may alert you and your doctor that something is wrong.

The other main type of persistent GTN is *choriocarcinoma*. In this condition, the molar pregnancy turns malignant, and it's more likely to grow and spread to organs outside of your uterus. You can think of choriocarcinoma as cancer of the placenta. Someone can develop this condition after a typical miscarriage, abortion, ectopic pregnancy or even a full-term delivery, but it's much more common after a molar pregnancy.

The risk of a partial molar pregnancy developing into choriocarcinoma is low — only about 1% to 5%. In a complete molar pregnancy, the risk of this cancerous-like spread is 15% to 20%.

The other types of persistent GTN, placental site trophoblastic tumor (PSTT) and epithelioid trophoblastic tumor (ETT), are even rarer. These tumors actually arise more commonly after typical deliveries or other nonmolar pregnancies, so I won't discuss them here.

Persistent GTN is treatable with chemotherapy, with a 75% to 95% cure rate. For people who don't want more children, removing the uterus (hysterectomy) is another effective option. Your doctor will talk to you about all your treatment choices.

When doctors can diagnose a complete molar pregnancy on ultrasound, they know there's a small risk that pregnancy tissue has already started to spread throughout your body (as an invasive mole or choriocarcinoma), even before you know that you've had a miscarriage. Cancerous cells can leave your uterus and travel in the bloodstream to other organs in your body.

The most common place that the molar pregnancy tissue spreads to is your lungs. A chest X-ray performed in the hospital, usually around the time of your procedure or before, can try to confirm that no tissue has spread outside the uterus.

My doctor told me that I needed to get a chest X-ray and lab tests before the procedure. Why was that?

Even if they're not spreading, molar pregnancies can have effects on other organs, so you'll also have blood testing to look at how your thyroid, liver and kidneys are functioning. This testing monitors for excessive thyroid hormone and preeclampsia, a potentially dangerous condition in pregnancy that leads to high blood pressure, liver inflammation and protein in your urine. Molar pregnancies can also cause ovarian cysts, so the ultrasound tech will examine your ovaries, too. I told you molar pregnancies were confusing.

TRYING AGAIN AFTER A MOLAR PREGNANCY

With most miscarriages, you don't have to wait before you can try to get pregnant again. But molar pregnancies are different.

That's because the only way that your doctor knows that you're safe from the risk of cancer with a molar pregnancy is to check your hormone levels. There is simply no other test that detects the spread of the placental tissue. And, unfortunately, that means that you should not get pregnant again after a complete mole until you've completed six to 12 months of blood tests. For patients with a partial molar pregnancy, most doctors want to see a weekly negative blood pregnancy test for one month before they stop the monitoring.

(?) YOU MAY BE THINKING ...

You're freaking me out with the word cancer. *Am I going to die?*

A molar pregnancy can be scary. Yes, tissue can spread and become choriocarcinoma, but not in most cases. The risk is low with a complete mole and incredibly low with a partial mole. The good news is that even if your hormone levels increased after the procedure, or your X-rays showed pregnancy tissue in your lungs or in other parts of your body, treatment with chemotherapy and possibly radiation can lead to a cure 80% to 90% of the time.

Thinking about cancer shows why it's important to get all the monitoring that the doctor thinks you need. If you're getting tested every week, your doctor will know right away if the levels are going up, which means that your doctor will be able to start your treatment immediately.

If you were to get pregnant again in the months after a molar pregnancy, your doctor wouldn't know if your pregnancy hormones increased because of the new pregnancy or because of the potentially cancerous old one. And in this situation, I would have to counsel my patient that I don't know if she just had a new pregnancy or if she has a new pregnancy and cancer. That's a situation no one wants to be in. As hard as it is to wait, the healthiest thing you can do for you and your future children is to monitor your hormone levels and put off pregnancy until your doctor gives you the all-clear.

Your doctor will talk with you about the kinds of contraception that are safest for you to use while you're waiting for the pregnancy hormone levels to drop. Your doctor will likely recommend that you use a highly effective method of birth control, such as an implant, injection or the pill. But if you don't want to or can't use hormones, talk to your doctor about barrier methods.

Doctors don't usually recommend intrauterine devices, because there's a higher risk of poking a hole in the uterus (uterine perforation) with an IUD insertion when you're healing from a molar pregnancy. But your doctor can give you information about your specific risks to help you make a decision about what contraception is right for you. If you don't feel comfortable using any form of contraception, it's vital that you don't have intercourse with a high risk of pregnancy until you get the green light from your doctor. Track your periods on a phone app, and don't have intercourse whenever you might be fertile.

Once you're in the clear, your chances of getting pregnant again aren't affected by a history of a molar pregnancy, though you have about a 1% to 2% chance of another molar pregnancy. But the other way to look at it is that 98 times out of 100, it won't happen again. It's likely, though, that your doctor will perform an ultrasound earlier than usual in your next pregnancy to make sure everything is progressing well.

✓ QUESTIONS TO ASK YOUR DOCTOR

Bring this list of questions regarding your options for treatment for molar pregnancy to your appointment.

☐ Why do you think this is a molar pregnancy?

_____

_____

_____

_____

☐ Where is the safest place for me to have the procedure done?

_____

☐ How often do I need to get blood tests?

_____

☐ Can I use a lab that's close to my home or work?

_____

☐ What are my best contraception options?

_____

_____

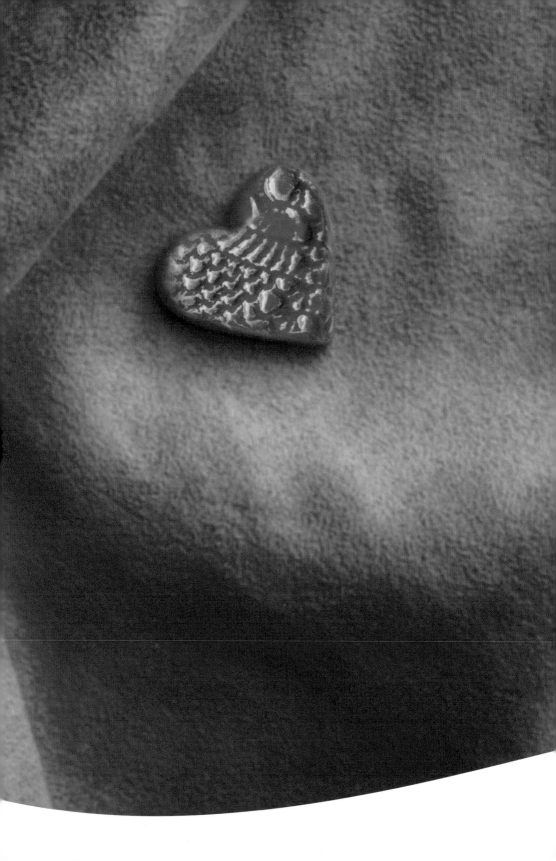

CHAPTER 12

Termination for maternal health reasons

I met Mina in the labor and delivery unit, where she had been admitted for severe high blood pressure at 22 weeks of pregnancy. Her doctors tried everything to lower her blood pressure, but her kidneys had started to fail, and she was at risk of heart failure and stroke if she stayed pregnant. The only safe choice for her was termination of her pregnancy. "I don't want to do this," Mina said to me, her eyes nearly swollen shut from crying. "But I have two kids at home, and I need to get back to them."

Pregnancy carries risks and uncertainty. It doesn't always end with a healthy baby in your arms, and many things can happen — from a premature delivery to losing your uterus or even dying. Doctors don't tell happy pregnant people this, as signing a consent form at your first prenatal visit acknowledging all the risks would put a damper on the whole "I'm pregnant!" feeling of joy. But the fact is, growing another human being inside of you impacts your health far beyond your uterus.

Sometimes pregnancy is a risk to your health after it's over — whether it's the effects on issues with your bladder, your blood pressure or even your blood sugar — but other times, pregnancy is truly unhealthy for a person during the pregnancy, even to the point of it becoming life-threatening. Being pregnant can create or worsen medical conditions that make it too danger-ous for you to continue the pregnancy. It's not something peo-ple think about in those early days of prenatal care, that their health might be adversely affected by trying to have a baby they want so very much. But to be a parent someday, or to be a healthy parent to the children that you already have, some-times means letting go of this particular pregnancy.

ⓘ MEDICINE-TO-ENGLISH TRANSLATION

These basic terms will be helpful for you to understand as you read through this chapter.

Dilation and curettage (D&C). A procedure of dilating (opening) the cervix and emptying the uterus of all preg-nancy tissue.

Dilation and evacuation (D&E). A two-step process of di-lating (opening) the cervix with medication or cervical dila-tors, and then removing the pregnancy and placenta.

Labor induction. The process of starting labor contrac-tions with medications to make the cervix open and deliv-er the baby and placenta.

Misoprostol (Cytotec). A medication almost always used in the medical treatment of miscarriage. Taken as multiple pills, it's swallowed, tucked in your cheeks (buccally) or placed in the vagina. Available by prescription, but not al-ways immediately available at the pharmacy. Often called miso for short.

People find themselves having to make these tough decisions because they either have a preexisting severe health condition or they develop a medical condition from the pregnancy itself.

PREEXISTING SEVERE HEALTH CONDITIONS

In some cases, your doctor may tell you as soon as you know you're pregnant that you shouldn't stay pregnant. Certain preexisting medical conditions risk serious harm to your health, or even death, while pregnant.

If you have one or more of the following medical conditions, it may be safer to terminate a pregnancy than to continue it:
- Breast cancer
- Cystic fibrosis
- Insulin-dependent diabetes with kidney damage (nephropathy), eyesight problems   (retinopathy), nerve damage (neuropathy), other vascular disease or of more than 20 years' duration
- Endometrial or ovarian cancer
- High blood pressure that can't be controlled (blood pressure that's at least 160 mm Hg systolic, the top number, or at least 100 mm Hg diastolic, the bottom number)
- HIV that's causing health problems or that's not being treated with antiretroviral therapy
- Reduced blood flow to the heart (ischemic heart disease) due to damage from a heart attack, infections, toxins or certain drugs
- Gestational trophoblastic disease (see Chapter 11)
- Hepatocellular adenoma, an uncommon and noncancerous tumor on the liver
- Cancerous liver tumors (hepatoma)
- Peripartum cardiomyopathy, a weakening of the heart muscle caused by pregnancy
- Schistosomiasis, an infection with a parasite that can lead to scarring (fibrosis) of the liver

- Uncontrolled seizure disorder
- Decompensated or severe cirrhosis
- Sickle cell disease
- Having a solid organ transplant (such as kidney, liver, heart or lung) within the past two years
- Stroke
- Systemic lupus erythematosus
- Genetic mutations that make it more likely that you'll get life-threatening blood clots (thrombophilia)
- Tuberculosis

You may need to see medical specialists to better understand your diagnosis and the health risks of these conditions during pregnancy. You might also see highly trained obstetricians called maternal-fetal medicine (MFM) doctors. No matter how many doctors you need to see, your team should make it very clear about your condition, give you information about your risks, and give you time and space to decide what to do.

One summer, my partners and I were referred two women for care. Both were recently diagnosed with breast cancer and were awaiting surgery to get a mastectomy. In the preoperative holding area, their routine pre-surgery pregnancy tests were positive. So the women had to have their surgeries canceled — since doctors are hesitant to operate on a pregnant person — and they were counseled to have pregnancy terminations before they could get surgery and chemotherapy.

It's difficult for me — or any doctor — to tell a person who wants a baby not to have one. It's equally hard to hear, especially if your condition doesn't make you feel sick! If you feel fine most of the time, you'd probably think, *How bad could it be if I got pregnant?* But that kind of wishful thinking leads to a lot of complicated and dangerous pregnancies.

I know I'm not supposed to be pregnant … but I really want to have this baby.

I totally understand that you may want a baby or another baby so desperately that you're ready to risk your own health to be pregnant. I don't think that the desire to become a parent, or to grow your family, is something to feel bad about. However, sometimes it's not until you're pregnant that the danger becomes frighteningly apparent. Doctors, who are professional worriers, are trying to avoid that exact situation for fear for your safety.

Admittedly, even if you had one or more risk factors for severe maternal health conditions, in some cases the pregnancy would turn out fine. No one can foresee the future with 100% accuracy. Boy, would I love to be able to tell my patients what the future holds for them and never be wrong.

So if you have one of these conditions, it's understandable why you would want to roll the dice. If that's the case for you, you'll need to find a doctor who will partner with you to get your health in the best shape possible before you get pregnant to give that pregnancy the best chance.

If a doctor tells you that you have a condition that under no circumstances should you get pregnant, it's reasonable to get a second opinion from another doctor. News like that is hard to hear, so it's OK to want to hear it twice or from a specialist to help you fully understand why pregnancy isn't possible for you.

PREGNANCY-RELATED HEALTH CONDITIONS

While your existing health conditions may raise serious questions about whether it's safe to continue a pregnancy, it's more typical for a new condition to develop during the pregnancy that puts your life in danger. These conditions aren't common, but I see them all the time in the large, urban hospital where I work. Let's go over these conditions one by one.

Preeclampsia

What used to be called toxemia, preeclampsia starts as early as 20 weeks of pregnancy. Doctors don't know what causes pre-eclampsia, though it seems to start in the placenta, where blood vessels don't develop or function properly. That's why it initially shows up as high blood pressure. However, it can progress from there, damaging organs like the liver and kidneys.

Anyone can develop preeclampsia, even if you've never had a history of high blood pressure. But it's more common in people with a history of high blood pressure or preeclampsia in previous pregnancies. Other risk factors include your age (very young or older than 35 years), obesity, race (Black), a twin or triplet pregnancy, a first-time pregnancy or conception through in vitro fertilization.

People don't always show signs or symptoms of preeclampsia, but the most common ones are:
- Blood pressure above 140/90 mm Hg on two occasions at least four hours apart
- Severe headaches
- Light sensitivity, blurry vision and temporary blackout of your vision
- Sudden weight gain or swelling in your face or your hands
- Pain in your upper belly, especially on the right side
- Nausea and vomiting, long after "morning sickness" should have resolved
- Trouble breathing

If your doctor thinks you're developing preeclampsia, you'll likely need to have a blood test and give a urine sample to look for:
- Protein leaking into your urine
- Decreased level of platelets in your blood
- Impaired liver function

Preeclampsia may begin with only high blood pressure. As it progresses and becomes severe, you can develop HELLP syndrome (which stands for hemolysis, elevated liver enzymes, low platelets). This is a sign that the disease is starting to affect your liver and bone marrow. And the scariest complication is eclampsia, when you start to have seizures.

The only cure for preeclampsia is ending the pregnancy, even if the pregnancy hasn't lasted long enough for the baby to survive outside of your body. Preeclampsia leads to severe complications when left untreated. In addition to HELLP syndrome and seizures, you're at risk of hemorrhage and stroke. It's simply not safe to let your pregnancy last any longer.

PPROM

If your water breaks too early in the pregnancy, which can happen in the second or third trimester, it's called preterm prelabor rupture of membranes (PPROM).When the baby is viable (usually around 24 weeks), PPROM can be managed with antibiotics and steroids to help the baby's lungs mature, and then inducing premature labor if infection develops.

But if your water breaks well before 23 to 24 weeks of pregnancy — the earliest time that most babies can survive outside of the womb — your risk of infection is high if the pregnancy isn't ended. An infection in your uterus isn't like a bladder infection that can be treated with antibiotics. Uterine infections can quickly spread into your bloodstream and threaten your life. Because the baby won't have enough time to continue growing and become able to survive delivery, doctors often recommend ending the pregnancy after your water breaks.

I know the thought of terminating a pregnancy is incredibly painful when the baby is still alive and appears to be healthy, but doctors haven't figured out a way to reseal the membranes after they break. Your doctor will be thinking solely about your health and ensuring that you will be healthy enough to have babies in the future.

Placenta previa

The placenta develops with the pregnancy to provide oxygen and nutrition to the fetus and removes waste from the baby. Think of it like a combination oxygen tank, feeding tube and trash disposal.

The placenta looks like a flat, round pillow that attaches to the wall of the uterus on its base and attaches to the baby via the umbilical cord. Most often, the placenta attaches to the top or side of the uterus. But sometimes, it implants very low in the uterus, where it partially or completely covers the cervix, which eventually needs to open for you to deliver the baby. This is known as placenta previa.

Your doctors may notice a placenta previa on ultrasound early in the pregnancy, and may reassure you that as the uterus grows, it will likely pull the placenta away from the cervix, and there's nothing to be concerned about.

However, if the placenta remains over your cervix as the pregnancy progresses, it can cause light and sporadic bleeding. "Pelvic rest" may help — no intercourse, douching or strenuous activity. But there's no way to move the placenta away from the cervix, or to "patch over" the part that's bleeding.

If the bleeding becomes heavy, you may need a blood transfusion. If it becomes very heavy or doesn't stop, it won't be safe for you to continue the pregnancy. If the baby is viable, your doctors will induce labor or, most often, perform a cesarean delivery. But if your baby isn't viable, your doctors may recommend terminating the pregnancy to preserve your health.

My doctors are telling me that I should stop this pregnancy because it's not healthy for me to continue it, but I've already told everyone that I'm pregnant. What do I tell people?

The news that something has developed with your health that threatens your pregnancy is devastating on so many levels. You're faced with a choice of having to choose the health of the baby or your own health. That choice is made all the more difficult by then having to potentially explain it to people.

If you had a condition before the pregnancy that your family knew about that is now threatening your health or your life, it may not be a surprise to them that it has now gotten worse and you may feel like you can be very honest with everyone. But if people don't know, revealing that you have a serious chronic medical condition is very personal, and you might not feel comfortable telling friends and co-workers about it.

It's your decision about what you choose to say or not say, whether everyone knows about your preexisting condition or not. If the medical condition developed during the pregnancy, it can be harder to know what to say.

The bottom line: Your doctors told you that you could die if the pregnancy continued, and for your own safety you had to stop it. Everyone who loves you should understand that choice.

TREATMENT

When it comes to treatment, terminating a pregnancy for the sake of your health looks very much like the procedures detailed in earlier chapters.

In the first trimester, you may have the options of medication therapy or a dilation and curettage (D&C). Using medication may be a possibility if the medical problem with your health is diagnosed and found to be severe early in the first trimester. Any medical problems that don't reveal themselves until later in the first trimester put you outside of the range of medication therapy, which means a procedure will be needed to remove the pregnancy. Depending on where in the pregnancy you are, your doctor may need to get your cervix ready with a medication called misoprostol (Cytotec), but the procedure and the recovery look the same as the D&C procedure for a miscarriage described in Chapter 6.

In the second trimester, you may have the choice between a surgical procedure or a labor induction. If seeing the baby and having a chance to say goodbye is important to you, labor induction is the way to go. If giving birth to a baby you can't take home would be even more painful, a dilation and evacuation (D&E) is a good choice. These are the same two options that people experiencing second trimester miscarriages have. Both are discussed in full detail in Chapter 7.

Make sure that your doctor explains to you clearly why terminating your pregnancy is recommended, what your options are for a second opinion, and how much time you have to make a decision. You may want to have the support of your partner, your best friend or your family during this time.

Even if your doctor conveys a sense of urgency, reach out to your support person to be with you when you're going through this — even if it's only by phone or video chat.

WHEN IT'S OVER

Physical recovery often takes days to a week or two. But the emotional recovery may take longer.

Feeling guilty is understandable. It's natural to feel helpless at not being able to protect your baby from the illness that's affecting your life. But a baby needs to grow inside of *you* — it's not in a vacuum, or a lab or an incubator. Doctors and engineers are researching how to do that — to be able to figure out how to have babies continue to grow when the uterus can't provide a safe home anymore — but science has not caught up to that need. In the end, if you're not healthy, the baby won't be either.

I want you to think about the importance of being healthy for the children that you have at home and being as healthy as you can be for the children that you're going to have someday. Even if right now you can't have this child, you need to be healthy first, before you can give life to another.

TRYING AGAIN AFTER A TERMINATION

Many people who terminate a pregnancy, for any reason, fear that their future pregnancies may be at risk. They worry that they won't be able to get pregnant again, even if their health improves, or that they are at an increased risk of miscarriage or pregnancy complications. Luckily, this is not the case.

Terminating a pregnancy under a doctor's care is incredibly safe both for your health now as well as for your chances of pregnancy in the future. An uncomplicated termination of pregnancy — even in the second trimester — does not change your future fertility. You will still be able to get pregnant just as easily as you could before, and your risk of another pregnancy complication is not higher. You'll have a recovery that's like one you'd have after a miscarriage, and you'll likely be able to try to get pregnant again as soon as you want to.

It is a fact backed by research that terminating a pregnancy — any pregnancy — is *always* safer than continuing one. And this is especially true for people facing the medical conditions discussed in this chapter. Please be careful about what you read on the internet. If you come across any information about the danger of pregnancy termination, bring it to a doctor who you trust. And if you ever feel that a doctor is not being honest with you, find another doctor.

✓ QUESTIONS TO ASK YOUR DOCTOR

Bring this list of questions to your appointment if your pregnancy is threatened by a medical condition. Take notes and check off the questions as you go.

☐ My medical specialist told me that the pregnancy is dangerous for my health. Do you agree? Why or why not?

_____

☐ Should I get a second opinion from another medical specialist?

_____

☐ Can I get a consultation with a maternal-fetal medicine (MFM) doctor?

_____

If you're struggling with a serious illness, the illness itself may pose risks to you now and in future pregnancies but terminating the current pregnancy does not. Talk with your medical team about taking some time to optimize your health before trying for another pregnancy.

☐ If I have preeclampsia, can my blood pressure be controlled in the hospital until the baby becomes viable?

_____

☐ If I have PPROM, can I be treated in the hospital until the baby becomes viable?

_____

☐ Do you think that surgery is a safe option for me, given my medical history?

_____

☐ Would you be the one to perform the surgery, or would it be someone else?

_____

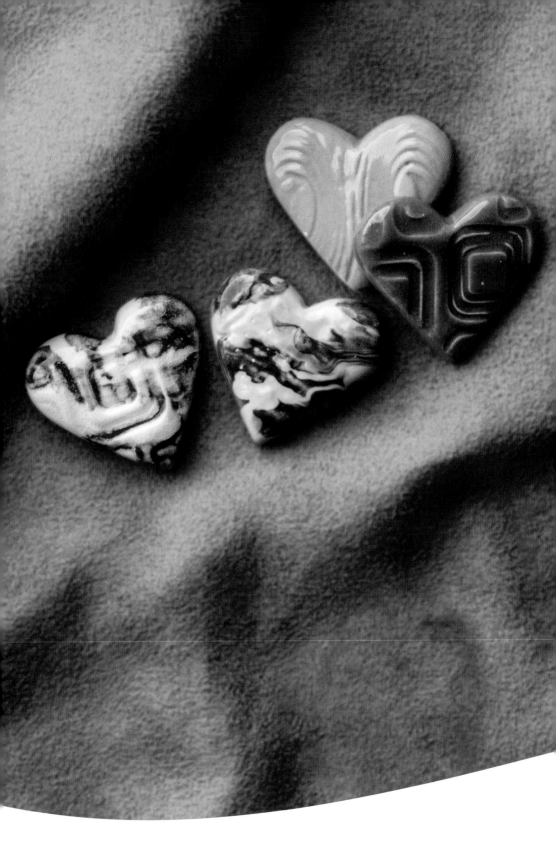

CHAPTER 13

Termination for fetal reasons

Nicole's genetic testing of her pregnancy revealed a lethal anomaly with the baby. When I asked how she was feeling, she bravely smiled up at me, and said, "Great."

But when I asked, "No, really, how are you doing?" she began to weep. Nicole talked about the fact that she stays healthy, really takes care of herself, has two beautiful healthy children, and never dreamed she would be in this position.

We've talked about pregnancy losses when the baby isn't healthy or developing normally. While typically these problems lead to a miscarriage early on, other problems don't. That means sometimes you'll make it into the second or even third trimester and then learn about a life-threatening or life-changing problem with the baby or the placenta. Genetic testing and ultrasound can detect a wide range of abnormalities with a fetus, from an extra finger on the hand or a cleft lip to bowel problems, heart problems or severe neurological problems. Sometimes the prognoses are clear, and it's known whether the problem can or can't be corrected after birth. However, sometimes a prognosis isn't clear and consultation with pediatric subspecialists is needed.

What to do with the news of a fetal problem is an incredibly personal decision. When faced with a baby that may have severe or lethal problems, some families choose to terminate the pregnancy, while others decide to accept what fate has given them for as long as the baby is alive.

ⓘ MEDICINE-TO-ENGLISH TRANSLATION

These basic terms will be helpful for you to understand as you read through this chapter.

Chorionic villus sampling. A procedure that removes a small sample of the growing placenta where it joins the uterus. Involves a long, skinny needle through your cervix or through your belly, using ultrasound as a guide. Used to test for chromosomal abnormalities.

Dilation and curettage (D&C). This procedure dilates your cervix and empties your uterus of all pregnancy tissue.

Multifetal pregnancy reduction. Reducing one or more of the fetuses in a multiple gestation (like triplets or quadruplets). Improves the chances that the remaining fetuses will be born healthy.

Radiofrequency ablation. A method of reducing a pregnancy with multiple fetuses. Uses a small needle device to send electric currents to interrupt the blood flow from your umbilical cord to one or more fetuses.

Selective reduction. Reducing a pregnancy with multiple fetuses when one fetus has an anomaly, or when a medical condition threatens the lives of one or more fetuses.

Another possible scenario involves pregnancy with multiple fetuses. One twin may be affected with an anomaly, or there may be a pregnancy complication that affects both twins' lives. If you're pregnant with triplets or even more fetuses, there are serious risks to the health of the pregnancy, even if the fetuses all appear to be healthy. In these situations, you may decide to reduce the number of fetuses to improve the chances of the remaining ones being born safe and healthy.

The last situation I'll discuss in this chapter is when you use a medication to manage a chronic medical or mental health condition that's not recommended for use in pregnancy … and then you become pregnant. The risk of a problem with the fetus may be high enough that the best decision for you and your family is to terminate.

DIAGNOSIS OF FETAL ABNORMALITIES

Fetal abnormalities are typically revealed at 11 to 13 weeks during the first trimester ultrasound or during the anatomy scan done between 18 and 22 weeks. Alternatively, doctors use blood testing, either at the end of the first trimester or in the middle of the second trimester, to detect abnormalities. At this point, you may be referred to a specialist to better understand your baby's condition. The specialist may recommend further testing, like an amniocentesis or an MRI.

Sometimes the medical team can't give you definitive answers about what kind of life your baby will have if he or she survives delivery. But the team should be able to give you the range of possible impairments — from mild, where the baby would need minimal medical intervention, to severe, which would require multiple procedures or a lifetime of therapy.

No matter the fetal prognosis, it's frequently an agonizing decision to consider terminating the pregnancy. People make all kinds of intensely personal decisions around whether to terminate a pregnancy with an abnormality. Some people feel that they have the resources to manage whatever difficulties their child will face. And if they feel that this may be their only chance at pregnancy, they may continue it no matter the odds.

But for many people, terminating a pregnancy with a serious condition is the best decision for the family that they have now, and the family that they hope to have in the future. But it's not an easy decision, even if you know the baby won't survive. And for many people, if they don't know for sure that their baby won't survive birth, they're not willing to take a chance.

For example, I've had patients who have one or more children with special care needs at home discover that they're pregnant with a fetus that's likely to have severe medical problems. Whether it's autism, a chronic illness or a birth-related complication, some children require a high degree of support. I tell struggling patients, "Love is infinite, but time, money and babysitters are not." These patients did not have the capacity to give birth to another child that would take resources away from their other living children.

Many kinds of abnormalities can affect a pregnancy. The most common ones I've seen are listed next; find links for more information on anomalies in the Resources section of this book.

COMMON FETAL PROBLEMS

The most common fetal abnormalities can be broken down into four types. Here's more on each type.

Chromosomal

Chromosomal problems can occur when there are too many

or too few chromosomes or when they are missing, duplicated or rearranged. Common examples of chromosomal abnormalities include:

Down syndrome (trisomy 21) An extra copy of chromosome 21 results in certain facial features and diminished physical and intellectual abilities. It may also be associated with heart problems and hearing loss.

Edwards syndrome (trisomy 18) An extra copy of chromosome 18 results in heart problems and abnormalities in the head and jaw. It's most often fatal in the first year of life.

Patau syndrome (trisomy 13) An extra copy of chromosome 13 causes severe intellectual disabilities, heart defects, brain or spinal cord abnormalities, very small or poorly developed eyes, cleft lip and palate, and weak muscle tone. It's most often fatal in the first year of life.

Gastrointestinal

A gastrointestinal abnormality occurs when the digestive tract doesn't develop properly, or the skin of the belly (abdomen) doesn't fully close around the intestines and other organs. Common examples include:

Duodenal atresia The upper part of the bowel is partially or completely blocked, which keeps the baby from being able to swallow and digest fluids.

Gastroschisis This is a defect of the belly (abdominal) wall next to the bellybutton. The intestines, and sometimes the stomach and liver, are found outside of the baby's body.

Omphalocele This defect of the belly (abdominal) wall causes the intestines and liver to poke out through the bellybutton. The intestines and liver are covered only by a thin, transparent sac.

Neurological

A neurological abnormality is the result of a problem with the development of the brain or spinal cord. These problems can often be detected on ultrasound at the end of the first trimester. Neurological abnormalities include:

Anencephaly This condition means the baby will be born without large parts of the brain and skull.

Caudal regression syndrome Abnormal development of the lower (caudal) end of the spine affects the spinal cord, bladder, bowels and legs. The symptoms it causes and how severe it is varies. Some babies have mild symptoms, while in others, this syndrome is disabling and life-threatening.

Dandy-Walker malformation This abnormal brain development affects intellect, movement, coordination, mood, and other functions of the brain and spinal cord.

Encephalocele A rare type of neural tube defect that causes part of the brain to poke out in a sac through an opening in the skull. Signs and symptoms include learning disabilities, growth delays, seizures, vision issues, uncoordinated voluntary movements (ataxia) and hydrocephalus, a condition in which a buildup of fluid in the skull puts pressure on the brain.

Holoprosencephaly With this abnormality, the brain fails to develop normally. It's associated with abnormalities of the brain and face, severe learning disabilities, and often seizures.

Spina bifida This lack of full development of the spinal cord can cause minor symptoms up to complete paralysis.

Structural

Structural abnormalities are problems with how a body part forms. They can affect a variety of structures in the body. These conditions range from mild to severe, but doctors aren't always able to say how severely a baby may be affected. Here are several examples.

Cleft lip and palate This lack of fusion of either the lip or the roof of the mouth can require multiple procedures over time to repair. Until the defect is repaired, babies have a very difficult time feeding and may not gain weight or grow the way they need to.

Conjoined twins This happens when identical twins are connected from the beginning of development to a degree that may involve just skin or the sharing of organs or limbs.

Cystic hygroma This fluid-filled sac, most often in the head or neck, is caused by a blockage in the lymphatic system. It can cause issues with the parts of the body it's near, including organs, nerves, blood vessels and the airway. Its effects vary from baby to baby.

Osteogenesis imperfecta This group of mild to lethal genetic disorders causes bones to break easily, often from mild trauma or with no apparent cause.

Renal agenesis (Potter's syndrome) This happens when the kidneys in a fetus fail to develop, causing a lack of fluid around the baby. As a result, the baby's limbs and lungs become deformed and impaired.

Tetralogy of Fallot This combination of four heart defects impairs the flow of oxygen to the body. A baby with this condition, especially if it goes untreated, may be at risk of serious complications and a shorter lifespan.

MEDICATIONS THAT CAN CAUSE FETAL ABNORMALITIES

There are two categories of drugs to be concerned about when you're pregnant or may become pregnant — Category D and Category X — and each has a different level of risk associated for use in pregnancy. These categories are being phased out, but your doctor may still use the terms.

(?) **YOU MAY BE THINKING …**

I asked my doctor about genetic testing for my pregnancy and he advised against it. He said, "You wouldn't want to have an abortion if you found something, right?" But maybe I would.

The biggest reason why most people want to have prenatal genetic testing is to find out whether the baby has a potentially serious or fatal condition. People want this information because they would prepare differently knowing it, such as delivering in a hospital that has special services, or because they might want to terminate the pregnancy, especially if the condition is very severe.

It's not your doctor's place to keep you from getting this information, and it's not up to your doctor to decide what you do once you have that information. That's up to you and your family alone. So if you receive awful news of an anomaly with your pregnancy, don't let your doctors' opinions of the "right thing to do" sway you one way or another. Get all the information you need, especially from a high-risk pregnancy doctor, a neonatologist or other specialist, and make the best decision for you and your family.

Category D medications

Category D medications have been shown to significantly increase the risk of fetal anomalies. However, you may need them to control a serious disease or prevent a life-threatening situation. If you're using any of these medications, talk to your doctor about the risks with pregnancy and if there are alternative options available. And if you become pregnant while using one of them, let your obstetrician know immediately.

Antibiotics that have been shown to significantly increase the risk of fetal anomalies include:
- Gentamicin, neomycin, amikacin sulfate (Arikayce Kit), streptomycin
- Trimethoprim-sulfamethoxazole (Bactrim, Septra, others) in the third trimester of pregnancy
- Nitrofurantoin (Macrobid, Macrodantin) in the past 36 weeks
- Doxycycline (Vibramycin, Doxy 100/200, others), minocycline (Minocin, others), tetracycline (Achromycin V)
- Fluconazole (Diflucan), voriconazole (Vfend)
- Primaquine, hydroxychloroquine (Plaquenil)

Neurological and psychiatric medications that have been to significantly increase the risk of fetal anomalies include:
- Fosphenytoin (Cerebyx), Phenytoin (Dilantin, Phenytek, others)
- Carbamazepine (Tegretol, others)
- Midazolam (Versed, others), alprazolam (Xanax)
- Phenobarbital
- Magnesium sulfate, though it's fine used during labor
- Lithium (Lithobid)

Heart-related medications that have been shown to significantly increase the risk of fetal anomalies include:
- Amiodarone (Pacerone, Nexterone)
- Atenolol (Tenormin)

- Lisinopril (Zestril, Prinivil, others), captopril, enalapril (Vasotec), benazepril (Lotensin)
- Losartan (Cozaar), valsartan (Diovan)
- Edoxaban (Savaysa)

Other drugs that have been shown to significantly increase the risk of fetal anomalies include:
- Cortisone, flunisolide
- Mycophenolate (CellCept)
- Penicillamine (Cuprimine, Depen)
- Methimazole (Tapazol), propylthiouracil, potassium iodide
- Hydroxyurea (Droxia, Hydrea, others)
- Tretinoin (Retin-A, Renova)

Category X medications

Category X medications pose an even greater threat to fetal development, so they're absolutely not recommended for use in pregnancy. As you'd do with Category D drugs, talk with your doctor about what the risk is to your pregnancy, and whether the possible abnormalities with the fetus are visible on ultrasound. After considering how a fetus might be affected by exposure to one of these drugs, many people decide to terminate their often very wanted pregnancy rather than take the risk.

Antibiotics that can threaten a baby's development include:
- Ribavirin (Virazole, Rebetol)
- Quinine (Qualaquin)
- Certain vaccines, including MMR (measles, mumps and rubella), shingles and chickenpox (varicella) within four weeks of conception and the TC-83 Venezuelan equine encephalitis vaccine

Heart-related medications that pose a threat to a baby's development include:

- Atorvastatin (Lipitor)
- Bosentan (Tracleer)
- Lovastatin (Altoprev)
- Pravastatin (Pravachol)
- Rosuvastatin (Crestor, Ezallor Sprinkle)
- Simvastatin (Zocor, Flolipid)

Skin (dermatological) medications that pose a threat to a baby's development include:
- Etretinate
- Isotretinoin (Accutane, others)
- Tazarotene (Tazorac, others)

Hormonal therapy that poses a threat to a baby's development includes:
- Danazol
- Megestrol (Megace ES)

Neurological and psychiatric medications that pose a threat to a baby's development include:
- Flurazepam
- Temazepam (Restoril)
- Triazolam (Halcion)
- Valproate (Depacon), divalproex (Depakote)

Other drugs that pose a threat to a baby's development during pregnancy include:
- Methotrexate (Trexall, others)
- Warfarin (Coumadin, Jantoven)

SELECTIVE REDUCTION OR MULTIFETAL REDUCTION

Doctors have long known that multifetal pregnancies increase risks to the health and life of both the pregnant person and the babies. The more fetuses present at one time, the greater the risks. For example, the risk of miscarriage of the entire pregnancy is 25% for quadruplets, 15% for triplets and 8% for twins. Even twin pregnancies, which have become more common in recent years thanks to in vitro fertilization and assisted reproduction, carry greater risk than solo ("singleton") pregnancies. Infants born after a multifetal pregnancy are at increased risk of being born early (premature); having cerebral palsy, learning disabilities, slow language development, behavioral difficulties, chronic lung disease, developmental delay, and vision and hearing loss; and dying.

When compared with singleton pregnancies, multifetal pregnancies are associated with a greater risk (five times) of stillbirth and an even higher risk (seven times) of dying in the weeks after delivery. Risks to the pregnant person carrying multiple fetuses include high blood pressure and preeclampsia, gestational diabetes, placental abruption and postpartum hemorrhage.

It's possible to perform a procedure to reduce the number of fetuses in the uterus, which lowers the risk of miscarriage and the other pregnancy complications to both the pregnant person and the surviving babies. The decision of which fetus to reduce is typically determined by technical factors, including the location of each fetus in the uterus. Selective reduction is a type of procedure where a fetus that has been diagnosed with an anomaly is the one that is reduced. On the one hand, these reductions improve the outcomes for the remaining fetuses. On the other hand, by its very nature, the procedure causes the loss of one or more fetuses. And in rare cases, it can cause a miscarriage of the entire pregnancy.

It's a complex decision to make. Patients must take into account the number of fetuses, their medical history, their values, and their particular economic and social situation. People considering pregnancy reduction may want to get input from many specialists before making their decision.

TREATMENT

The same procedures outlined in earlier chapters are the ones used to terminate a pregnancy for what's called fetal indications — because of a problem with the baby.

In the first trimester, you'll likely need a dilation and curettage (D&C) to remove the pregnancy. Fetal abnormalities aren't generally diagnosed early enough for medical management. Depending on where in the pregnancy you are, your doctor may need to get your cervix ready with a medication called misoprostol (Cytotec), but the procedure and the recovery look the same as the D&C procedure that's described in Chapter 6.

In the second trimester, you may have the choice between a surgical procedure or a labor induction. If seeing the baby and having a chance to say goodbye is important to you, labor induction is the way to go. If giving birth to a baby you can't take home would be even more painful, a dilation and evacuation (D&E) is a good choice. These are the same two options that people experiencing second trimester miscarriages have. Both are discussed in full detail in Chapter 7.

Multifetal pregnancy reduction most often takes place in the first trimester but can also occur in the early part of the second trimester. Often doctors will recommend a procedure called chorionic villus sampling (CVS) to confirm that the remaining fetuses are genetically healthy.

The reduction itself may happen in a doctor's office or in an operating room. The most common procedure is performed using ultrasound as a guide. Your doctor will insert a thin needle into your belly or vagina, into the pregnancy sac, and inject a special drug into the fluid surrounding the fetus. This medication, potassium chloride, quickly stops the fetus's heart.

For "higher order multiples"— where there are four or more fetuses — the doctor will repeat the procedure to reduce the pregnancy to twins or triplets. Sometimes, a technique called radiofrequency ablation will be used instead. This is when a small needle device uses electric currents to interrupt the blood flow from your umbilical cord to one or more fetuses.

Whichever procedure is used, the doctor will perform an ultrasound to confirm that the other babies still have a healthy heartbeat. Some people are able to go home after the procedure; others stay in the hospital overnight for observation.

Make sure that your doctor explains to you clearly why you are getting this diagnosis, what your options are for a second opinion, and how long you have to make a decision about whether or not to terminate the pregnancy. This process may be one that you want to do with your partner, your bestie or your family. Even if your doctor conveys a sense of urgency for you to decide, reach out to your support person to be with you when you're going through this — even if it's only by phone. And for the procedure itself, try to have someone by your side so you're not going through it alone.

(?) **YOU MAY BE THINKING ...**

I don't think I could give birth to a baby that would be seriously sick or possibly die. My husband and I know that's the right decision for us, but how do we explain this to other people?

Sadly, in America, terminating a pregnancy is no longer a personal choice, but a political one. I wish that this decision, which is so hard for people and their families, could just be made in private and be respected by everyone. But many of us know people, sometimes in our own families, who would not understand such a decision.

For family or friends who you think would be supportive of your need to make a decision like this, I encourage you to be honest with them. This can be an excruciating time for you and your partner, and you need all the support you can get.

But for people who have ardent anti-abortion views, it's not your responsibility to enlighten them. It may be easier in some cases to simply tell these people that the baby died rather than make yourself vulnerable to heartless judgment after such a complicated decision.

RECOVERY

Physical recovery often takes days to a week or two. Infections from these procedures are rare. After multifetal reduction, there is a small risk of miscarriage and of preterm labor. You may need more visits with your doctor and possibly more ultrasounds than usual to check on the health of your babies.

But the emotional recovery from a decision like this may take longer. It's common to feel torn or guilty about your decision. You may be faced with a situation in which there is no good answer, and nothing feels right.

I want you to take comfort in the fact that you are being the best parent you can be. If you have children at home, you are doing everything you can to parent them in the best way you know how, which includes ending this pregnancy. And if you don't have children at this time, you did right by this pregnancy in the best way you could.

TRYING AGAIN AFTER A TERMINATION

Many people who terminate a pregnancy, for any reason, fear that their future pregnancies may be at risk in some way. They worry that they won't be able to get pregnant again, or that they are at an increased risk of miscarriage or pregnancy complications. Luckily, this is not the case.

Terminating a pregnancy under a doctor's care is incredibly safe both for your health now as well as your chances of pregnancy in the future. An uncomplicated termination of pregnancy — even in the second trimester — does not change your future fertility. You will still be able to get pregnant just as easily as you could before. You'll have a recovery that's like one you'd have after a miscarriage, and you'll likely be able to try to get pregnant again as soon as you want to. You may want to have a genetic counsel-

PREGNANCY SHOULD BE A PRIVATE MATTER

Terminating a desired pregnancy is a brutal experience. The pain of this decision can be compounded by the reactions of other people in your life. Sometimes my patients feel compelled to lie, sometimes to their closest family and friends, to save themselves from criticism and judgment.

It really is no one's business why you're making the choices that you're making, but once a pregnancy is public, people very often feel that they have the right to comment. Unfortunately, being pregnant is a public act, and people feel more comfortable than they should telling a pregnant person how they should and shouldn't eat, drink or live, just because they're pregnant. This extends to having opinions about what people should do with the pregnancy when there's a problem.

Let me be clear: It's none of their business. They're not you, and they don't have to live in your reality. I don't care how many miracle stories other people have read on their Facebook feed about babies that survived at a ridiculously premature age or were born healthy when the doctors said they wouldn't be. You and your family should make the best decision you can with the best information that your medical team can give you.

ing consultation to talk about what the chances are of the anomaly recurring in a future pregnancy. You might also want a preconception visit with a maternal-fetal medicine specialist to talk about early diagnosis options in your next pregnancy. Take time to gather all the information you need to make the best decision you can about trying for pregnancy in the future.

✓ QUESTIONS TO ASK YOUR DOCTOR

Bring this list of questions with you to your appointment. Ask about your options for a pregnancy complicated by a serious condition with the fetus. Take notes and check off the questions as you go.

For a fetal condition:

☐ What is the range of possible outcomes of this condition?

_____

☐ Can I see a pediatric specialist to talk about the diagnosis?

_____

☐ Is it possible to get a referral to a children's hospital?

_____

For a medication that can cause abnormalities:

☐ How soon could we see the problem on ultrasound?

_____

☐ Can I get a second opinion with another ultrasound?

_____

☐ Can I get a consultation with a maternal-fetal medicine doctor?

_____

☐ What is the range of possible outcomes for the baby?

_____

For selective reduction or multifetal reduction:

☐ How do you figure out which fetus(es) to reduce?

_____

☐ Can we perform testing on the fetuses to help make that decision?

_____

☐ Would you be the one to perform the procedure, or would it be someone else?

_____

☐ What are my options for anesthesia during the procedure? Can I be fully asleep?

_____

☐ What are the risks to the remaining fetus(es) of this procedure?

_____

_____

_____

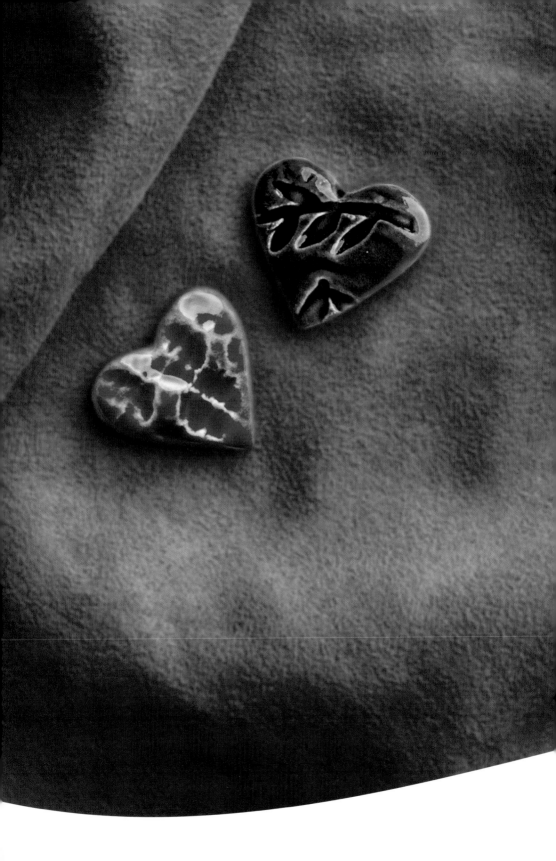

CHAPTER 14

Ambivalence and loss

Olivia made an appointment for a medical termination of her unplanned pregnancy. When the doctor told her that the embryo didn't have a heartbeat and that she'd had a miscarriage, he thought she would be thrilled. Instead, Olivia froze. "What happened?" she said, crying. "What's wrong with me?"

Society doesn't leave much room for people who aren't jumping for joy at the idea of being pregnant. As little as miscarriage is talked about in public and in movies and TV shows, people hide ambivalence around pregnancy even more. Many resources around miscarriage assume that you grieve the loss. But the diagnosis of pregnancy leaves many people, frankly, shellshocked. Once that initial surprise fades, you may feel very confused and unsure.

THE NORMAL (AND WIDE) RANGE OF EMOTIONS

Here's a secret that OB-GYNs know: Feeling uncertain about an unexpected pregnancy is almost as common as is miscarriage itself. You may have felt uncertain about an unexpected pregnancy in the first place or feel ashamed for having mixed feelings about your loss. But the truth is that even though most people publicly say they're overjoyed to be pregnant, many feel a range of emotions, including the following.

Completely surprised

If you're using birth control or having sex infrequently, you may be shocked that you're pregnant. If you have a history of infertility or have had difficulty getting pregnant, getting pregnant "on your own" may be confusing. If this current pregnancy comes soon after another, you might also be surprised that you were able to get pregnant again so quickly. Or you might be shocked if you thought you were too old to get pregnant.

Financially concerned

Whether it's your first or fifth baby, you may not be sure how you're going to afford this baby or what you're going to do for child care. You may wonder how being pregnant and going on parental leave — if that's even an option — will affect your career. You may not know how you're going to make room for another person in your current home, or not know how you can afford a bigger place.

Medically scared

If you're struggling with a medical condition, you may not know what it means for your health to be pregnant. And if you're on medications for this condition, it can lead to a sinking feeling in your stomach when you find out that you're pregnant. This is especially true if doctors have told you that you shouldn't be pregnant while taking these medications. You may remember that you had a drink (OK, a lot of drinks) in what would have been the first few weeks or months of your pregnancy, when you didn't even know you were pregnant. Now you're scared that you hurt the pregnancy.

Worried

Being pregnant and having a baby leads to changes in so many things — your body, your relationships, your life. It leads to change for other children you may have. Some of my patients are afraid that their partners will leave them — or worse, hurt them — once they find out about the pregnancy. And not being sure how you're going to handle all these changes is normal.

Inadequate

If you had trouble bonding with, breastfeeding or comforting one or more of your previous infants, or you have been struggling with parenting in general, you might view a new pregnancy with fear or uncertainty.

Alone

It can be isolating if your partner or family is excited about your pregnancy, but you're not feeling the same way. Or if you don't have a partner, or if your partner is deployed overseas or working out of state, the prospect of single parenthood may be daunting.

Unsupported

People don't hold back from judging pregnant women. Whether the pregnancy is one you wanted or not, everyone has an opinion — about how old you should be when you get pregnant (which is not too young and not too old), about how you

WHEN 2 BECOME 3

Having a baby changes the dynamics of every relationship. You may be terrified of all the ways that a baby will forever change your relationship with your partner, now that you may become parents. It's possible that your partner isn't feeling the same way you are about the pregnancy. Maybe your partner can't be around very much due to work hours or because you live apart. Perhaps your partner is ambivalent about becoming a parent or becoming a parent again if there's already another child in the picture, either with you or with another partner. Maybe your partner isn't "into" babies and has already said that taking care of an infant is off the table. Or your partner doesn't want to take any time away from work or hobbies when you bring the baby home. I've heard all of this and more from my patients.

Even though this pregnancy may have ended in a loss, it has likely brought up a lot of feelings in both of you. You may want to consider a heart-to-heart conversation with your partner about pregnancy, as part of your recovery. Talk about what the prospect of a baby means to both of you — what your thoughts are about parenting a child together, when might be the right time, what goals you want to achieve before bringing a baby into the picture. Use this as an opportunity to grow close together in planning your future together.

should behave when you're pregnant, about what you should and shouldn't drink and eat, about the place you'd be bringing the baby home to. … If they see you as struggling in any way, some people don't hesitate to cast judgment on you or even state outright that you shouldn't bring a baby into this world.

Women who are chronically ill or struggling with substance use disorders face even harsher judgment, perceived as selfish for wanting to have a baby. It's a double stigma, daring to want to be a parent while still fighting the disease of addiction.

Wanting to become a parent is one of the most natural things in the world. That desire doesn't always consider how sick you are, if you're struggling, or if you're young or old. The heart wants what it wants. So if family or friends are not validating your feelings, speak up. Let them know how you are feeling, and that while the miscarriage may look like a good thing to them, it is breaking your heart and you need their support.

Traumatized

If this isn't your first pregnancy, you may have strong emotions about a previous pregnancy or loss. You might recall the sleep deprivation you experienced with your last baby, the lack of help from your partner, or the postpartum depression you experienced. Knowing what might lie ahead after delivery can be a source of more pain than comfort.

Anxious or depressed

For people who experience anxiety or depression or have in the past, an unexpected pregnancy can make symptoms worse. If you're on medication to help manage these conditions, that also brings up a whole host of questions about whether you should keep taking them, knowing that you desperately count on them to keep you functional and well.

Confused

Part of you may be feeling excited about the prospect of a baby, but part of you knows that now is not the right time, or that you're not with the right person, and you're conflicted about how you resolve these different feelings. You may even be too afraid to tell anyone that you're pregnant while you're trying to figure out what to do.

Worried about the changes to your body

You have every right to have mixed feelings about the changes in your body, which might feel foreign. Even people who are excited to be pregnant have told me that it feels like having "an alien inside" them or that they feel "possessed" by the growing baby. And if you rely on your body for your career, as models and athletes do, you may wonder if you'll be able to "get your body back" after giving birth.

Terrified of childbirth

You also may be scared by horror stories of childbirth. Well-meaning (or sometimes not well-meaning) family, friends and acquaintances gleefully may recount for you how horrible their birth experiences were. Stories about strangers' experiences in childbirth are just a few clicks away. My unofficial tally is that there are more scary stories on the internet than there are reassuring ones.

Frightened of postpartum depression

You might be worried about developing postpartum depression. It's heartening that so many women and even celebrities feel comfortable about sharing their experiences with depression after childbirth. But hearing these stories can give you one more thing to worry about when you're thinking about having a baby. And if your mother confided in you that *she* struggled with postpartum depression, your risk is higher — which may leave you even more concerned.

Overwhelmed by what comes after

You may be concerned about what it will be like to bring the baby home. You may not be excited about being home alone with a newborn all day. If you're being honest with yourself, you may not feel like you're a baby person, even if you like kids in general.

Even if you plan on going back to work, it's possible that you'll be home for 2 to 3 months by yourself with a baby. You may be worried about bonding with this new being who you are responsible for taking care of. Or worry about feeling angry or resentful that a baby — no matter how cute he or she is — is a bundle of needs 24/7. You may already get cranky when you stay up too late binge-watching television or stay out at a party well until the wee hours. You may worry about how you'll function with a newborn at home.

Unsure about parenting *at all*

Some people may not be sure if they ever want to parent. Many of my patients feel that the prospect of becoming a mother or father is something they *should* want, rather than something they *do* want.

It's becoming more common for people to assert that they don't want to have a child. I'm heartened that more and more of my patients say that they need reliable birth control methods for the rest of their childbearing years or even that they want to be sterilized young because they know they don't want to have children. But this bone-deep certainty about not wanting to become a parent doesn't stop the pressure from family or friends or society in general about having a baby. No shortage of people will try to convince you that you will regret it later in life if you don't have a baby, though generally those same people don't ever engage with you.

YOUR FEELINGS DIDN'T CAUSE YOUR MISCARRIAGE

Whew! No wonder not all people know what they want to do when they find out that they're pregnant. Being diagnosed with a miscarriage while they're deciding what to do about the pregnancy doesn't make it any easier. Books and blogs and even your doctor may assume that you are grieving the loss and that sadness is your major emotion. But the mixed feelings that many people experience about an unexpected pregnancy are just as common with miscarriages.

Even if you didn't want to be pregnant, a miscarriage can be devastating. And that can add even more confusion. You may think, *I wasn't happy about being pregnant, so why am I so sad that it's over?* Some people decide to terminate the pregnancy and then are shocked when it's a miscarriage, like my patient at the start of this chapter. Some may feel shame or guilt at being relieved that they're no longer pregnant, even though there was a long list of reasons that the circumstances weren't right. Others may have decided to continue the pregnancy despite their circumstances and then feel guilty when it's a loss, as if in some ways their reluctance caused the miscarriage to happen.

You may be really surprised by your complicated feelings. But the same worries will come for you as they do for people with a welcomed pregnancy: not knowing what this means about your body or your health or whether you'll have pregnancies in the future. Even if you weren't sure that you wanted to have a baby right now, it's nice to know that you're healthy and could have a baby if you wanted to.

A miscarriage isn't a punishment for anything that you thought or how you felt or what you did. Your guilt did not cause your miscarriage. We talked about all the things that don't cause a miscarriage in the very first chapter and I want to make this point crystal clear: **Your ambivalence did not cause your pregnancy loss.**

No matter how many of the emotions in the list you just read rang true for you and no matter what you lie in bed at night worrying over, *you did not make the miscarriage happen.* Think about it this way: If willing a miscarriage into existence was as simple as not wanting the pregnancy (even *really* not wanting

---

(?) YOU MAY BE THINKING …

I really wasn't sure how I felt about being pregnant. I honestly think I'm happy that I'm not pregnant anymore. Does that make me a bad person?

It's OK if relief is one of many feelings that you're having — or even the main one. If it was going to be a hard decision about what to do with the pregnancy, you may feel grateful that the choice was taken out of your hands. If you knew that now was not the most ideal time in life to be pregnant and have a baby, a miscarriage can be a good thing for you in the end. I've had many patients call a miscarriage "a blessing" because, as they put it, it was like their body or God or the universe knew what they couldn't handle it and made the decision for them.

Human emotions are messy, and "all the feels" are normal. If you are taking any comfort in your miscarriage, see it as a positive, and not one more thing to feel guilty about.

---

the pregnancy), then there would be many fewer abortions every year. You can't control what happens to your pregnancy any more than the people who are thrilled beyond belief to be pregnant can. So while you're untangling the thicket of emotions you may be feeling, please know that all these feelings are normal, even if you weren't sure you wanted to be pregnant at the start. And know that this outcome was in no way a result of what was in your heart.

✓ SELF-REFLECTION AFTER A LOSS

You may feel a whole host of emotions in the days and weeks after your loss. As time passes, you may want to reflect on some of the things that came to the surface after you found out you were pregnant.

☐ If you have any health concerns, do you need to see your doctors to work on getting healthier for a possible pregnancy in the future?

_____

☐ If you have any financial concerns, do you need to think about a plan to get into a more secure situation before another pregnancy? Can your partner or family help?

_____

☐ If you haven't talked with your partner about having babies, do you want to begin that conversation?

_____

☐ If you know you don't want to face pregnancy in the near future, do you want to talk to your doctor about your birth control options?

_____

☐ If pregnancy brought up feelings of anxiety or depression, do you want to talk to a therapist to work through those feelings?

_____

☐ Do you want to think seriously about if you ever want to parent at all? Or if you want to parent more children in the future?

_____

_____

_____

PART 4

Healing

After a diagnosis of pregnancy loss, there's a flurry of activity — tests, appointments, procedures, more tests, more appointments. But once the miscarriage is over, there's often … silence. After the medical concerns fade away, the hard work of grieving and healing begins.

This part of the book addresses the many physical feelings and emotions you may experience. You'll also have an opportunity to reflect on how other people in your life experience your miscarriage. Finally, this section ends with ways for you to remember the pregnancy.

CHAPTER 15

What to expect when you're no longer expecting

Pilar sat silently as I gently discussed her options for how to proceed with her 14-week miscarriage. We talked about her options and I stressed that she didn't have to decide that day. She asked softly, "How will I feel this weekend once the baby is gone?" I knew she didn't mean just how her body would feel.

People react to death in many kinds of ways. Your upbringing, culture and personal experiences with illness and death influence how you respond to loss. People experiencing miscarriage can land anywhere on the wide spectrum of grief, and their feelings can change moment to moment. At the same time, your body is still recovering. How you feel emotionally and how you feel physically may feel one and the same — lousy — or you might feel a disconnect between the two.

You can go back and forth between feeling at peace and like you are moving on ... and then feeling down and tired and not being sure why. As a doctor, I want to tell you that however you experience grief is OK. Having a mixed bag of feelings during this time is completely normal. There is no one way to get through the grief of a miscarriage. My patients have felt all of these things — and so have I with both of my losses.

In the first days and weeks after miscarriage, you may feel:
- Sadness and pain
- Disbelief and numbness
- Anger and outrage
- Helplessness and guilt
- Isolation and loneliness
- A yearning for the baby
- A need to talk about the baby or the miscarriage
- A need to *not* talk about the baby or the miscarriage
- An urge to cry all the time
- Concern for your partner or your other children
- Fear of future losses or of not being able to get pregnant again

People experiencing pregnancy loss report feeling all those emotions. Research has shown that miscarriage typically causes significant distress — much more than many doctors or the public realize. In fact, the feelings of distress, trauma and grief can be just as deep and challenging as they are after losing a loved one.

You may feel anxious and uncertain about a range of physical and emotional issues. Let's discuss some of the concerns that my patients have most often expressed.

GOING HOME

If you were admitted to the hospital for your miscarriage — generally in the second or third trimester of your pregnancy, or if you experienced complications in the first trimester — you might feel that staying in the hospital will help you recover more quickly. It can also be reassuring to have doctors and nurses around.

A generation ago, people routinely stayed in the hospital for a week or more after having a baby, and it wasn't much different after a miscarriage or stillbirth. But doctors learned that being in the hospital — when you don't need the acute level of nursing care that comes with it — can make it more difficult to recover.

If your doctor is worried about your bleeding or you are being treated for an infection, you may stay in the hospital for a few days. But otherwise, the best place for you to heal is at home. There, you'll sleep better and ideally be surrounded with people who love and care for you. You'll have your own food and your own shower and a lot less noise when you're trying to sleep.

Shouldn't I stay in the hospital longer? It feels like I'm being discharged home too quickly.

Once you're home, the most important thing to do is to listen to your body. Take it easy and avoid activities that cause pain. Try to get back into your routine as quickly as you can, as getting up and about can speed your recovery. Eat what you want to, shower or bathe as you usually do, and exercise, if that's a regular part of your life.

BLEEDING AND YOUR NEXT PERIOD

It's common to worry about post-miscarriage bleeding and how long it will last. Most people bleed for 2 to 3 weeks after a miscarriage. This depends on whether you had a procedure or were treated with medications. Bleeding typically lasts longer after expectant or medication management than after a procedure. You may have all kinds of bleeding patterns in that time — bleeding heavily at first and tapering off over time, bleeding on and off, or bleeding like a period for weeks.

As soon as the bleeding stops, you may wonder about your next period, which should happen anywhere between three and six weeks later. The further along in pregnancy you were, the heavier that first period is likely to be. Be sure to stock up on pads or tampons.

STILL FEELING PREGNANT

After pregnancy loss, your body parts can be out of sync with each other. Your hormone levels slowly return to normal, despite the sudden loss of the baby. Typically, the nausea and fa-

---

THE BABY STUFF

One of the many decisions you'll face in the days after your loss is what to do with the baby things that you may have been given or bought in preparation for birth. If you were far along in the pregnancy, you may have an entire room painted and furnished and ready for a baby. You may have had a baby shower and have a pile of presents awaiting thank-you cards. On the other hand, you may have purchased only a few things.

Like everything else about miscarriage that's discussed in this book, there's no right or wrong answer regarding what to do next. If you can't bear the thought of coming home from the hospital to baby gear and gifts, your partner or your bestie can pack things away before you're discharged. If you don't have storage space in an attic or basement, perhaps a family member would be able to hold things that would cause you pain in the coming weeks. You may want to be the one who decides what to put away and what to keep handy. Don't assume that your partner or your family know what you want — let them know what you're thinking.

tigue resolve first, in the first three days after the miscarriage is over. If you were in the second or third trimester, your back and joints will need time to recover.

Breast tenderness is the last thing to improve, as the high progesterone levels that cause this discomfort take the longest to adjust. Your breasts may leak milk, especially if your pregnancy loss was in the sec-

I started leaking milk from my breasts today— what's happening?

If you have the baby's room ready, you may agonize over what to do next. Make no decisions in the first days when you're home, and only go into the room if you want to. When you're up for it, see how the room makes you feel. If the sight of an empty crib makes you feel horrible, perhaps pack the furniture away. Consider how it feels best to use the room — for remembering the baby, like a chapel as a place of prayer or meditation, or as a quiet room for thinking about the future. But if the nursery makes you feel hopeful about someday bringing a baby home to it, leave it just as it is, as a testament to both the baby you lost and the one that hopefully awaits you in the future.

I had bought a pair of baby overalls the day I got pregnant for the first time, and they hung on my dresser until I was hospitalized when I lost the baby. My husband, Chad, thought the sight of them would be too painful for me, so he put them in a drawer where I could easily find them but didn't have to see them when I wasn't ready. This thoughtful act was exactly what I needed.

ond or third trimester. The hormonal shifts after delivery lead to milk let-down and discomfort in your breasts as they swell. You can help reduce how much milk your body produces by wearing a tight-fitting bra (such as sports bras), refraining from any stimulation of your breasts, and facing away from the water in the shower, since heat can cause more milk let-down.

As for weight gain, I tell my patients that it takes as long to lose pregnancy weight as it did to gain it. So if you were four months pregnant when you had your miscarriage, don't expect to lose the pregnancy weight in any sooner than four months. One of the many injustices of pregnancy loss is that you may still look pregnant for a few weeks afterward.

SEX

It's natural to want to be close to your partner when you're feeling emotionally wrung out. Traditional advice holds that you should refrain from intercourse for two weeks after the loss to allow the cervix time to close and reduce the risk of infection. Although this advice is not based on research, I tend to be conservative in my advice around sex — the better-safe-than-sorry approach.

But this doesn't mean you shouldn't orgasm. In fact, I highly encourage it, if you're feeling up to it. Sexual activity can be a life-affirming way for you and your partner to come together after the miscarriage. And I'm all for the healing power of the release of endorphins and hormones that come with orgasm.

It's also natural to not feel ready for intimacy after your miscarriage. Your body may be physically healing from the loss, especially if you needed surgery, and you're likely still bleeding. Beyond the physical aspects, it's understandable to be cautious of sex — it could lead to a pregnancy that you're not ready for or that reminds you of the baby you lost.

PREGNANCY LOSS WITHOUT A PARTNER

This chapter assumes that you have a strong support system around you — a partner, family and friends. I want to take a moment to talk to the strong people managing this loss on their own or with a partner who is unsupportive or with a partner they aren't emotionally close with.

Like other losses, miscarriage can be hard to get through alone. You often need physical comfort — I'm a strong believer in the therapeutic power of a hug — and someone to process your feelings with. This support doesn't need to come from a life partner. For many of my patients, it comes from a mother, sister, cousin or best friend.

Don't hold back from reaching out to the people who care about you. In many cases, they'll be glad to be able to actively help you by being present, by listening or even by late-night texting. Ask them for food, for companionship, for funny memes — whatever gets you through the initial period of physical recovery and beyond.

Friends and family, by blood or by choice, aren't your only resources. Check out support groups at your hospital, seek out friends of friends who've had miscarriages, or visit online communities (see the Resources chapter). These are all potential sources of support. You may be surprised at how miscarriage creates a bridge between strangers who may have had different journeys but find themselves grieving in similar ways over the same kind of loss.

If you have a partner, talk about how you are feeling. Try to stay physically close, if that brings you comfort, in ways that aren't sexual. Hand-holding, cuddling and back rubs are all examples. And if you're not a touchy person by nature, let your partner know other ways to offer support right now. Give yourself time to feel in control of your body again before thinking about sharing your body with someone else.

OTHER CONCERNS

While concerns about staying in the hospital, post-miscarriage periods, still feeling pregnant and intimacy are common, they may be just the first of many concerns you may have. Here are some other things my patients routinely say they're feeling. You may be experiencing these feelings, too.

"This was my first pregnancy. I just can't get over that this happened to me."

You never think that a miscarriage is going to happen to you, especially when you're young or a pregnancy comes at the right time and with the right person. So you may feel like your body is broken or has betrayed you in some way. To see that body unable to hold a pregnancy shakes up your entire self-image around what your body can do. And when it's your first pregnancy, a miscarriage often shatters beliefs about your body. You may wonder if you're going to ever be able to have a baby. These worries about the future are common and largely overblown, as most people who miscarry go on to have healthy pregnancies afterward.

"I feel torn apart, like I'm physically and emotionally missing a piece of myself."

Many people from the earliest moments of the pregnancy picture the baby taking first steps, riding a bike, graduating from high school and sometimes even getting married. Even though the baby doesn't progress beyond being an embryo or fetus, that early mental picture of a child, teenager or adult remains.

Pregnancies can represent hope and optimism and plans for the future, not only for the pregnant person but for the entire family, and that's a lot of thoughts and feelings wrapped up as what begins as a simple cell. This pregnancy may be "just" an embryo, but to you it may feel like an entire life. The loss of a pregnancy is a loss of all the hopes and dreams that go along with it, so it's no wonder it can feel so horrible.

"I have other children. Why am I so despondent about the loss of this one?"

Just as every child is different, every pregnancy is different. This pregnancy represented a new journey, a new set of hopes and dreams. You may have been thinking about how great your other kiddos would be as big brothers or sisters to your new addition to the family. You might have had a picture in your mind of what your new family would look like, or how you planned to space your children's ages. Even when you've borne a healthy child or healthy children, and you know your body can do it, there is still a genuine sense of loss.

"People are telling me that it was early in the pregnancy, so I shouldn't be this upset."

People are dense. Grief is not proportional to gestational age. Research shows no association between the duration of the pregnancy and the intensity of grief. Pain cannot be measured by a ruler or a calendar.

People are well-meaning, but they often say the wrong things (see the list of "Rotten things people may say to you" on page

260). Do not let anyone else tell you how you should feel. Your grief is going to progress in its own way and at its own time. Don't let anyone make you feel judged for how that process happens.

"One day I'm fine and thinking about trying again, the next I'm weeping in the grocery store."

You'll likely have good days and bad days. Small things — sometimes literally, like seeing baby socks or baby shoes — can trigger an emotional reaction. Or it might be hearing the name you had picked out for your baby, or a "Congratulations, Mom!" from someone who didn't know about the loss. For me, a "My Mama's for Obama" onesie in a store window led to a full-on crying meltdown on Sixth Avenue in New York City.

Anything that reminds you of the pregnancy, and your future hopes and dreams, can make the grief come back in a big wave. This is a typical part of coping with loss.

"This feels like a loss I'll never get over."

When you lose someone who you love — a parent, a good friend or a child, including a pregnancy — you can feel like the pain will never go away. And in the throes of grief, you may feel like you're never going to be happy again. For now, know that these despairing feelings are normal. In the next chapter, I'll talk about what to do if these feelings don't leave you after a few weeks.

"I feel like I've let everyone down."

One of the worst parts of grief, I think, is guilt. Guilt for not conforming to what others expect of you, for not giving your parents the grandchild they wanted, even for not feeling worse about your loss. Especially if you're a people-pleaser much of the time, you may feel bad for the other people who are disappointed by your pregnancy loss.

Try to recognize that the miscarriage was out of your control, and no one should blame you for the loss. You're all feeling the pain together. I'll talk more about this in Chapter 16.

"I'm thinking weird thoughts and I don't want to tell anybody, especially my partner."

Are you hearing a baby cry? Especially when you're home or at night? Especially if you lose a pregnancy later in gestation, it's not unusual to hear babies crying. You are not losing your mind. Do you feel like you're still pregnant? To this day, if I notice my breasts feeling heavy, or have a bout of gas that feels like a baby kicking, it can take my breath away.

Thinking that you hear a baby or still feel pregnant or other bodily feelings around the pregnancy may make you feel odd, but they're normal. You don't need to see a psychiatrist. That said, if your weird thoughts involve harming yourself, **please seek help immediately.** Reach out to your doctor or go to an emergency room or call a suicide hotline. In the U.S., the **National Suicide Prevention Lifeline** is **1-800-273-8255**.

"My family is treating me like they think I'm going to fall apart. Is it wrong that I'm doing kind of OK?"

In the same way that grief is a part of life, so is healing. Unfortunately, everybody else may want to project their feelings onto your situation. It's possible that your family and friends aren't seeing exactly what you're feeling but are responding more to their fears about you or their own feelings of grief.

You may need help managing everyone else's feelings. Sometimes people get in the position of comforting people who come to them crying about the loss, and you find yourself in the position of, "Why am I giving *you* a hug? I'm the one who lost a baby here."

If you find yourself with well-meaning and loving family and friends coming to you too much with their own feelings of grief, feel free to appoint someone — whether it be a sister or best friend or your partner — who can help keep these people at bay until they feel better. If that's not possible, you may need to be direct with them about how you need them to manage their grief without heaping it on you.

Try saying something like, "I'm slowly healing from this loss, and I feel better each day. But it makes it harder for me when I hear about how much you're suffering. I know you're hurting for me and my loss, and that you want the best for me. The best way you can help me is to be strong in front of me, even if that's not always how you feel."

"I have the opposite problem — no one is taking my miscarriage seriously."

Society fails miscarriage, whether that's from lack of awareness, cultural norms of individualism, or deciding what kind of relationships deserve to have children. Heartless or clueless people may try to deny you the grief that is rightfully yours, especially if you're a teenager, unmarried, in a same-sex relationship, transgender or someone else not universally deemed as worthy of having a baby.

Know this: **You are a parent, even if your baby did not survive until birth.** You became a parent the day you found out you were pregnant. You have every right to grieve this loss. Repeat this to yourself whenever you need to.

In addition, surround yourself with people who will support you and validate your loss. If you don't have a good support network near where you live, or at all, it can be helpful to seek out local support groups and online communities. Ask your doctor for a referral to the hospital social workers, as they are often the ones with the best knowledge about what is available in your area.

"I'm starting to feel good again — and I feel horrible for feeling good."

It is *so* normal to feel guilty when you're feeling good. In your mind, you may have expectations around how long your period of mourning should last, or feel that in some ways, if you stop being sad, it means that you don't miss the baby. But grief has no set timeline.

Starting to feel good again doesn't mean you're forgetting about the pregnancy or that you don't have feelings. Whatever you're feeling about your pregnancy loss is OK, including starting to be able to let go of your grief. Consider this your permission slip to feel whatever you want to feel and forget about what everyone else thinks.

"Honestly, I've been doing OK all along. Is that wrong?"

Absolutely not. Not everyone sees a pregnancy loss, especially one in the first trimester, as a life-altering event. Some people recognize that the odds of miscarriage mean the future most likely holds a healthy pregnancy for them. If that's you, then it's completely fine to not be completely whipsawed by grief. In the same way that I want to validate the grief around the miscarriage, let me validate that feeling OK is equally normal. There is no right or wrong way to manage a pregnancy loss, and I for one am glad that you're taking it so well.

ROTTEN THINGS PEOPLE MAY SAY TO YOU ... AND WHAT THEY NEED TO KNOW

Even well-meaning people can say lousy things in their attempts to comfort you. This list offers just a handful of things that have been said to my patients or to me.

Check off all the things that have been said to you or people you know, and write ones in the margin that I've missed.

☐ You can try again.

☐ You'll get pregnant again.

☐ You should be grateful. You already have one child.

☐ You can always adopt.

☐ This is God's plan for you. It was God's will.

☐ Everything happens for a reason.

☐ Time heals all wounds.

☐ At least you know you can get pregnant.

☐ It wasn't meant to be.

☐ At least it was early in the pregnancy.

☐ You're stressing too much.

☐ Thank goodness you have your health.

☐ There was something wrong with the baby anyway.

☐ It happened for the best.

☐ At least you're young. You can try again.

☐ You're too old to have a baby anyway.

☐ At least you didn't really know the baby.

☐ It's not like losing a child who has lived with you.

☐ I know exactly how you feel.

Here's what I want to tell these (probably) well-meaning people:

- No comfort follows the words "At least."
- Stop looking for the silver lining or any version of "looking on the bright side."
- You need to mourn *this* pregnancy.
- You wanted *this* pregnancy.
- This may have been your only or last chance at pregnancy.
- Children are not interchangeable. Having a child at home does not diminish the loss of this pregnancy.
- All losses are worthy of grief, no matter how early in the pregnancy.
- No one can ever know exactly what a grieving person is going through.
- Referencing a future pregnancy is *spectacularly* unsupportive.

"I lost my baby at the end of the first trimester, but my friend had a stillbirth at eight months. I feel like her grief must be so much worse than mine, like I don't even have a right to be sad when I'm around her."

There is no cosmic contest around grief. You can always find someone who's had more loss than you have. Just because someone else is experiencing grief — the magnitude of which may look enormous to you — does not mean that you can't feel grief, too. There's nothing to be gained by comparing your pain to anybody else's, and that goes in both directions.

I mentioned how researchers haven't been able to find an association between the length of gestation and intensity of grief, anxiety or depression. Yes, someone who experiences a stillbirth at eight months will probably be devastated. But so may a person undergoing in vitro fertilization whose transferred embryos didn't take. That's a loss, too.

You might be tempted to think you were pregnant for "only" a short time, but your pain is just as valid as somebody else's. It's just a reminder of how many people are in this community of having undergone loss around pregnancy. You have more in common than you realize.

⊘ QUESTIONS TO ASK YOUR DOCTOR

Bring this list of questions to your appointment so you can ask what to expect in the first days and weeks after your loss. Take notes and check off the questions as you go.

☐ How soon should I see you in the office after my miscarriage?

_____

☐ How long should my bleeding last?

_____

☐ When should I go back to work?

_____

☐ When do you think it's safe for me to have sex again?

_____

☐ If I want to talk to someone about the loss, can you give me a referral?

_____

☐ Does the hospital have a support group for people with pregnancy loss?

_____

_____

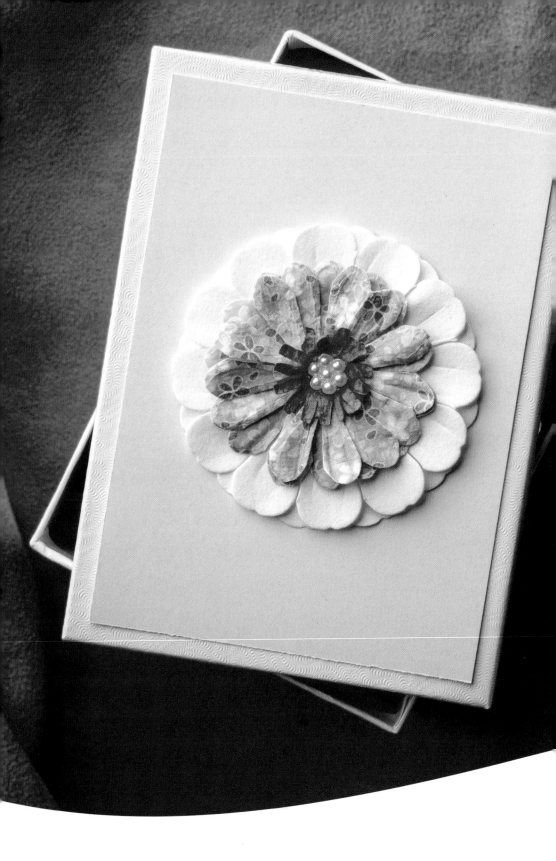

CHAPTER 16

Managing your grief

Quinn, a 27-year-old mother trying for her second child, sat on the exam table after her second pregnancy loss. Wiping away tears, she said, "I don't think I can go through this again. I can't sleep. I can't eat. It's hard to breathe. I don't know how to get through this."

The last chapter addressed the emotional roller coaster of reactions to miscarriage. In this chapter, I'll explore what grief after pregnancy loss might look like in the months after a miscarriage and how to recognize when grief transforms into something more serious.

Right away, I want you to know that if you're feeling in free-fall crisis mode and you flipped to this chapter first, **it is OK and necessary to get help.** Reach out to your partner or to a health care provider you trust. Ask for an urgent appointment, and if you can't even wait that long, go to the emergency room. Trust me when I tell you that you would not be the first person after a loss to come to the emergency room because you're at your wit's end and you don't know what to do.

Take care of yourself before taking care of anyone else. Make sure that right now, in this moment, you are OK.

GRIEF AFTER LOSS

After your loss, you may experience months of highly intense emotions. Some people may experience all these feelings, others just a few. Sometimes you proceed through these emotions one at a time, and sometimes you jump around, feeling one emotion one day and another the next. And on exhausting days, you may flip back and forth before bedtime. Here are some of the most common emotions you may experience.

Denial

You may feel numb at first and be in total shock when you get your diagnosis. I've had patients ask for two, three or even four ultrasounds to prove to them that the heart of the baby is no longer beating. It can be so difficult to accept that the pregnancy is truly over, especially when you still feel pregnant.

Sadness

Sadness is the biggest emotion that people think of after a loss. You may find yourself crying all the time, especially if crying is a way that you cope with big emotions. It certainly is for me, and I was quite soggy for a long time after my losses.

Sadness may be expressed as yearning for the child you lost; this emptiness might even feel like a physical pain. For some people, sadness may be not so much yearning as feeling incomplete. A miscarriage has been described as not losing an entirely separate person, but as losing a part of yourself.

Search for a meaningful explanation

There's a stage when you can become completely preoccupied

with the loss, asking *why* over and over. Needing to find an answer for the miscarriage can dominate your thinking. You may have trouble focusing on anything else. Your sleep patterns may change, ranging from being unable to sleep to sleeping for long periods of time. Your eating habits may change, too — you may lose your appetite, or you may end up eating much more than usual. This can even result in noticeable weight loss or gain, depending on how long this state lasts.

Anger

You may feel angry at the unfairness of the loss, especially if you felt like you did "everything right." You might be angry at your doctor or midwife, who you think might have been able to stop the miscarriage from happening if he or she had just done *something*. Anger may come out at your partner or your children because it can be less painful to feel anger than to feel sadness. You may even be angry at yourself, blaming yourself for not being able to stop the loss.

(?) **YOU MAY BE THINKING ...**

Everybody thinks I should be "over it" by now. But I don't want to be over it.

It's not unusual to want to hold on to the pain of the miscarriage. It may feel like surrounding yourself with the pain is the only way you can still hold on to the baby. The sadness and thinking about the baby make the pregnancy still seem real in a way, and to let go of the sadness feels like letting go of the baby. In Chapter 18, I'll talk about healthy ways to memorialize the pregnancy.

Guilt

Guilt is an expression of underlying self-blame. Guilt was one of my most painful issues to work through in therapy. I felt that my first job as a mother was to keep my baby safe, and I utterly failed to do this. And because I had medical trauma associated with my first loss, I was overtaken by guilt as to why I survived when my daughter didn't. Guilt has been found to be the strongest — I would say the most insidious — aspect of grief after pregnancy loss and needs time to resolve.

Bargaining

Bargaining is common with any kind of grief. You may find yourself making bargains or promises to God, to fate or to the universe to get the baby back or make sure that your next pregnancy is healthy.

Acceptance

The intensity of these feelings will eventually wane. Most people begin to accept the loss and can settle back into life as they know it. This doesn't mean, though, that the loss isn't always a part of you. Some of my patients describe it as a piece of their heart or a part of their soul that always bears the wound of the miscarriage. It may not seem like it now, but that part does get smaller with time.

Acceptance can take longer than you would expect. It can take up to six months or a year after the loss, and some experts think even up to two years after the loss, before you feel like you've regained your balance.

Bottom line: There's no set amount of time that is "normal" to grieve a loss of any kind, including a pregnancy loss.

Delayed grief

Some people experience delayed grief, where their first intense feelings are brief. Emotions may simmer until rearing up around six months, and then they start to ease. This pattern is typical for people who are working hard to "hold it together," but grief can seldom be denied, just delayed.

Grief is normal

The bottom line with grief is that it's a process, and this tiring toggling between emotions is to be completely expected. Your ability to cope with your feelings will be strong on some days, and not so good on others.

Grieving for a long time is less of a concern than is the intensity of your grief. I tell my patients to think not so much about the calendar as about how their grief affects their lives. If your grief impacts your work, your relationships and the rest of your life, you could benefit from some help, even if it hasn't been "that long." Without help, grief can turn into adjustment disorder, where you feel symptoms similar to depression and it takes you up to six months to feel like yourself again.

If your feelings interfere with your ability to live your life the way you want to for more than two weeks after your miscarriage, it's a good idea to talk to your doctor. Even if you're not sure if you need help, the two of you can discuss it.

POST-MISCARRIAGE DEPRESSION

Even when a pregnancy is going well, many people worry. It's normal to feel some anxiety about the baby or the pregnancy. And it's normal to have mixed feelings about the changes that the pregnancy is bringing to your body and your life right now, as well as all the changes it will bring after the birth. Especially if you're prone to worrying, pregnancy gives you many great reasons to feel nervous. And research shows that a person is more at risk of emotional illness during and after a pregnancy compared with other times in life. So, it's not surprising that when that pregnancy ends at a loss, you risk de-

---

(?) YOU MAY BE THINKING ...

Everybody thinks I shouldn't be this sad after an early miscarriage.

I've said before in this book that there is no ranking of pain, and no person has any more right than another to feel upset about a pregnancy loss. But people who lose a baby in stillbirth or shortly after birth have familiar rituals, like funerals and memorial services, that provide comfort and a public structure for people to support them.

However, when people have a miscarriage early in pregnancy, or even a failed in vitro fertilization (IVF) cycle, the loss can feel invisible and unresolved. Because you weren't showing, the pregnancy may be less real to the people around you than it was to you. While other people who love you may have been sad that you lost the pregnancy, if it never seemed as tangible to them, they may have a hard time understanding why you still feel the way you do.

Don't let anyone pressure you to cycle through your grief stages any faster than you think you need to. All pain is valid, even if other people don't understand it. Stand in your truth, and your pain, regardless of when you miscarried. And take all the time you need to get whole again.

veloping depression. A family history of depression, lack of support or any additional stress — like a job change, moving, serious illness of a loved one, or even spending the holidays with your family (if they're less than harmonious) — all increase your risk of post-miscarriage depression.

Research shows that major depression is more common in women who've had a miscarriage than in those who haven't been pregnant. And if you've had depression in the past, a miscarriage may trigger a recurrence. Of all women who've ever been depressed, up to half will become depressed after a pregnancy loss. And if you don't think you can confide in your family or friends, you get the perfect setup for grief to slide into depression.

It doesn't matter how far along you were in the pregnancy, how old you are or even how you felt about the pregnancy. Brain chemistry and pregnancy hormones interact in ways doctors don't completely understand, but this link between miscarriage and major depression is real.

Grief versus depression

When your grieving process seems unbearably intense or persists for a long time, you may have prolonged or complicated grief. Or it may be an indication that you're now experiencing depression. It can sometimes be hard to tell the difference, especially when you're in the middle of it. Timing alone doesn't always provide clarity. Prolonged grief can be diagnosed as soon as six months after your loss. But "regular" grief can last for more than six months without being deemed abnormal. One thing is certain: Grief has to have a significant impact on your daily functioning before it can be diagnosed as prolonged grief.

One way I put it to my patients is this: Crying and deep sadness are OK, but a lack of coping and deep despair to the point that you're not taking care of yourself is not. It's the difference between weeping in the shower ... and not taking showers at all. Or between deeply missing the baby ... and wishing you had died as well. I've had patients become so overcome with grief that they spend 18 hours a day in bed, essentially stop eating, or are unable to interact with the rest of their family at all, including their young children.

If you continue to feel debilitated by your emotions or your feelings of sadness seem relentless, this is when I would worry. If your feelings of depression persist beyond several weeks and begin to interfere with your ability to function at home or at work, it's time for professional support. Your doctor can help figure out whether you have major depression or are experiencing prolonged grief. And you and your doctor can decide together what is the best way to get you help.

There are people who experience depression after a miscarriage that feel such deep guilt, shame, self-doubt or sadness that they have thoughts of hurting themselves. So it's incredibly important to know when you need to seek help.

If you feel like your sorrow just isn't lifting in the way that you hoped it would, your doctor may use a two-question screening test for depression to assess how you're doing. This test is called the Patient Health Questionnaire-2 (PHQ-2), and it asks the following:

Over the last two weeks, how often have you been bothered by the following problems?
• Little interest or pleasure in doing things
• Feeling down, depressed or hopeless

For each question, give yourself zero points if you answer, "Not at all," 1 point for "Several days," 2 points for "More than half the days," and 3 points for "Nearly every day." If you score a total of **3 points or more,** it doesn't mean that you have depression, but your doctor should perform a full evaluation to see if you meet the criteria for any of these disorders.

And if you don't score 3 points or more but are still concerned about how you're doing, read on to the next section.

Warning signs to watch for

When depression does occur, it can last for 6 to 12 months after the miscarriage and sometimes longer. Depression is *always* something that you should talk with your doctor about. If you're not sure whether to seek help for your feelings, ask yourself these questions.

☐ Do you feel you're not coping well with your miscarriage?

☐ Are you not able to sleep or get out of bed?

☐ Do you find yourself turning away foods, even those that you love? Or do you find yourself eating constantly, unable to stop? Have you noticed that you've gained or lost more than a couple of pounds?

☐ Are you not keeping up with everyday self-care, such as getting dressed, bathing and preparing food?

☐ Do you feel like the amount of worrying or nervousness or tension that you have is worse than it should be?

☐ Can you not watch an entire television episode or read a magazine article or book chapter without losing focus? Do you lose concentration in conversations with other people?

☐ Have you had any difficulty caring for your other children or keeping up with household responsibilities?

☐ Are you lacking family, close friends or a partner supporting you through this?

☐ **Most important of all:** Are you having any thoughts of hurting yourself or someone else, even if they're just vague thoughts without a plan for how to do so?

If you answered **yes to any of these questions,** please reach out to your doctor to talk about these issues. It can be hard to reach out when you're feeling this awful, but that's what your doctor is for — to keep you safe not only during the miscarriage, but also afterward.

Treatment for depression

Depression is treated with talk therapy, medication or both. Talk therapy involves speaking with a licensed mental health professional who can help you process what you're feeling. This professional can give you ways to manage your thoughts so that you can function properly again. Medication therapy involves taking antidepressants, which help many people feel like themselves again.

Which treatments you use depend on what symptoms you have, how intense they are, how often they occur, how your symptoms impact your everyday life, and what other medications you're taking.

No doctor should push you into accepting a treatment you're not comfortable with. But even short-term therapy or medication can give you your life back.

ANXIETY AND POST-TRAUMATIC STRESS

Miscarriage triggers high anxiety, and not just for worrywarts.

In fact, anxiety symptoms may be even more common than depression symptoms after miscarriage. Almost half the people experiencing pregnancy loss will show symptoms of anxiety, which centers on pregnancy-related issues.

It's normal to worry about developing physical problems after a dilation and curettage (D&C), like continued bleeding or vaginal discharge. It's normal to worry about possible underlying medical illness that contributed to the loss. Many people fear whether they'll ever be able to have a baby and are anxious about the prospect of another miscarriage. They spend enormous amounts of mental energy agonizing over the trauma and trying to determine why it happened. From here, some spiral into guilt, blame and shame. And the less support you have to lean on, the more likely it is that you'll feel anxious.

One loss can create fear of other losses. Many people who have a miscarriage become suddenly afraid of losing everything from their phone and their keys to meaningful relationships. You may even feel as if you're losing your faith or any hope of the future. While it's normal to fear losing what's important to you, please reach out to those who love you for additional support.

Although anxiety symptoms are widely common after miscarriage, it's less clear what the risk is of developing an anxiety disorder. Research suggests that in the first month after pregnancy loss, about a quarter of people have symptoms consistent with moderate to severe anxiety, and even more have symptoms of post-traumatic stress. These symptoms improve over the first year after loss but can be more intense for people who experience ectopic pregnancy.

When do the "normal" symptoms of post-miscarriage anxiety become a disorder? Like with depression, anxiety becomes a disorder when the symptoms are difficult to control and interfere with everyday functioning. Here are a few examples, with descriptions to help you recognize them.

Acute stress disorder

Acute stress disorder (ASD) may affect 1 in 10 women who has experienced a miscarriage, and the symptoms can begin within hours of knowing you've lost the pregnancy. The symptoms of ASD include numbness or lack of emotional responsiveness, and persistently feeling edgy or in distress. You may be unable to recall events that happened around the miscarriage, such as receiving the diagnosis or what the procedure was like.

The miscarriage makes me feel like I could lose anything, and I feel panicky all the time.

Post-traumatic stress disorder

Conversely, you may relive the loss through recurrent thoughts, dreams or flashbacks. Post-traumatic stress disorder (PTSD) is when these symptoms last longer than a month, unlike with ASD, in which the symptoms resolve within four weeks.

Generalized anxiety disorder

Less severe but equally distressing is generalized anxiety disorder (GAD). You might be diagnosed with GAD if you experience persistent and excessive worry on most days, for more than six months, and you have additional symptoms. In addition to persistent and excessive worry, you may experience:
• Restlessness or edginess
• Extreme fatigue
• Troubles with concentrating or remembering things
• Irritability
• Muscle tension and aches
• Sleeping problems

- Digestive issues
- Rapid heartbeat

The simplest screen for anxiety disorders is called the General-ized Anxiety Disorder 2-item (GAD-2). Like the depression screen on page 272, there are two simple questions:

Over the last two weeks, how often have you been bothered by the following problems?
- Feeling nervous, anxious or on edge
- Not being able to stop or control worrying

For each question, give yourself zero points if you answer, "Not at all," 1 point for "Several days," 2 points for "More than half the days," and 3 points for "Nearly every day." If you score a total of **3 points or more,** your doctors should perform a full evaluation to see if you meet the criteria for any of these anxiety disorders.

MOVING FORWARD

When you're experiencing normal grief, most often the inten-sity of your symptoms will decrease over 6 to 12 months. After this initial period, though, you'll likely experience spikes of intensity during certain events. Some of these occasions are predictable, but some may take you by surprise.

The next pregnancy

You *will* heal, even if it doesn't feel like it today. And you may decide to try to get pregnant again. Some people feel that when they think about another pregnancy, it somehow betrays the memory of the one they lost. But being ready to move on to the next stage of your life, whatever that is for you, isn't a sign that you've forgotten the other pregnancy. Feeling strong again and looking toward the future and what it might hold doesn't mean you've erased what's happened to you in the past.

If you want it to be, this pregnancy will always be a part of you. You don't need to keep grieving a miscarriage to respect the baby you lost. You can be happy with a new pregnancy and still terribly miss the pregnancy that wasn't meant to be at the same time. The happiness of the new does not replace or kick out the old. You can hold both in your heart at the same time.

MANAGING INTRUSIVE, PAINFUL THOUGHTS

In the darkest days of my life after my first pregnancy loss, I routinely experienced flashbacks to the trauma that surrounded the loss. It wrecked my concentration and kept me awake at night. Telling myself to think of different things was useless. Thankfully, my amazing therapist shared a visualization technique that has stuck with me, even more than 10 years later.

She talked me through how to stop a painful thought, recognize and validate it, and picture placing it on a conveyor belt and watching it roll away. This worked for the worst memories, but for those of my daughter, it was too painful to watch thoughts "leave." Instead, I visualized myself placing those thoughts in a white satin box — the same kind of memory box I was given in the hospital — and then onto a shelf in a mental closet. This process helped control the intrusive thoughts without making me feel like I was letting go of them completely. I still feel like I can open that white box in my mental closet whenever I want, and whenever I'm ready to do so.

It is important to note, though, that people who have had a rough time healing after a pregnancy loss are more likely to feel depressed in the next pregnancy and experience postpartum depression. It's not unusual for these feelings of guilt or sadness to come back again unexpectedly. Tell your doctor that you have a history of miscarriage so that you can receive better mental health care in your next pregnancy.

The anniversary of the loss

It's common to have an *anniversary reaction* after a pregnancy loss. It can happen around the day you found out you were losing the pregnancy, perhaps the day of the ultrasound that showed no heartbeat or the day you began bleeding. It also might be the baby's estimated due date. It's not uncommon for people who have been feeling well and healed to suddenly feel sad again, to belatedly realize that the day on the calendar holds some significance for that pregnancy.

You may want to tell your closest friends or family that you're anticipating a rough time around a particular date, so they can be sensitive to what you may be feeling. You may plan around these dates, especially in the first year after a loss. That means no high-pressure situations and no obligations that require a lot of concentration — unless you think that they may provide a distraction. For me, it's Feb. 22, the day I lost my first pregnancy. I try to take that day off from work when possible, because I know that I may be in tears before the day is over.

The out-of-the-blue triggers

Unexpected events can also unleash in you a strong emotional response. I certainly didn't expect to lose it when I saw that "My Mama's for Obama" onesie in the store window. For some people, it may be a holiday you pictured celebrating with your baby. For others, it might be hearing the name that you chose for your baby, even if it is just a character in a movie. Even now, television shows or movies that show a baby dying (really, Hollywood?) or a child in peril can upset me for days.

Sometimes, you may expect to be fine at a celebration such as a baby shower. You plan for it, you steel yourself for cute baby things overload, and you don't expect to be surprised. One of my dearest friends who suffered a second trimester pregnancy loss of a boy attended a baby shower for her sister-in-law. She had plenty of time to prepare for the event but was gobsmacked when her other sister-in-law gave the expectant mother a family heirloom. The gifting sister gave the present with the words,

THE BABY SHOWER FOR SOMEONE ELSE

Accepting someone else's pregnancy, and even feeling genuinely happy for the parents-to-be, doesn't mean it will be easy to sit through a party celebrating it. Receiving an invitation to a baby shower when you may still be grieving your own pregnancy loss can feel like a knife to your heart. Acknowledge the mixed emotions (you're allowed to have them) and give yourself some time to figure out what you feel ready to do.

If you want to attend the shower:
- Visualize in advance what may happen during the party — comments about how radiant the pregnant person looks, conversation about childbirth and newborns, pink and blue everywhere. This may prepare you for the sights and sounds of the event.
- Consider making an appearance but not planning to stay the entire time if you're feeling unsure about at-

"My son had this, and I want your son to have it." When she realized that this gift likely would have been given to her son had he lived, my friend needed to flee to the basement, weeping, to compose herself. She hadn't thought to prepare for this gift exchange, and it felt like a sucker punch.

The pregnancy of a friend or family member

A dreaded situation comes up when friends, family members or co-workers announce pregnancies of their own. You can hold two feelings in your heart at once — that you're incredibly happy for them, and that you're sad about your own loss.

tending. Have an excuse ready that will allow for a graceful exit.

- Attend with a friend who knows what you're going through, if possible — someone who can give you a hand squeeze or crack a joke if you appear to be struggling.
- Similarly, have an exit strategy if you find yourself overwhelmed by emotion. You can convey congratulations to the pregnant person's mother or partner, and quietly slip away from the celebration.

If you don't feel ready or able to go to the shower, *that's OK, too*. There is no rule that you must accept every party invitation you're given, even if it's for a family member or close friend. You can still express joy and congratulations with a heartfelt card and gift, presented on your own time in a way that doesn't require putting on a brave face in a roomful of people.

It's human to feel jealous, too, and to wonder why pregnancy is succeeding for them when it didn't for you. I tell my patients that it's better to acknowledge these feelings rather than ignore them. When you're alone or with your partner, acknowledge your feelings and feel free to curse an unjust universe.

Luckily, there aren't a finite number of babies in the universe. Accept that someone else's pregnancy does not take away your pain or reduce the chance that you, too, will have a healthy pregnancy someday. By processing these feelings in a safe space, you'll be in a better state of mind to manage your emotions and allow you to be there for your loved one.

Support groups and counseling

Research shows that talking to other people who have experienced miscarriages provides the strongest support. These people have a better chance of understanding the emotions you may be feeling. You may find that they seem to understand you even more than do your closest loved ones if your loved ones haven't experienced a miscarriage themselves.

There are many ways to share your story with other people. While therapy tends to be one-on-one, many kinds of group sessions and web-based forums bring people and couples together with a common history of miscarriage or pregnancy loss. Sharing your story, whether it's with strangers on web-based forums or through group sessions, can make you feel less alone and more understood. Sharing your experience also gives you the opportunity to help others who may be earlier in the grieving process than you. Sometimes nothing makes you feel as good as helping someone else start to feel better.

> I think I need to talk about this because my partner doesn't seem to understand why I'm so upset.

Your doctor can help you find a grief counselor, and your hospital may have a loss program for families. Look in the Resources chapter of this book for online communities and other organizations dedicated to helping people and couples manage pregnancy loss.

✓ QUESTIONS TO ASK YOUR DOCTOR

Bring this list of questions to your appointment to ask your doctor about managing your grief. Take notes and check off the questions as you go.

☐ How long am I going to feel this way?

_____

☐ How can I better manage my anxiety?

_____

☐ How can I tell if I'm becoming depressed?

_____

☐ Do you know about local resources for people coping with pregnancy loss?

_____

☐ If I want to talk to a therapist, can you refer me to one?

_____

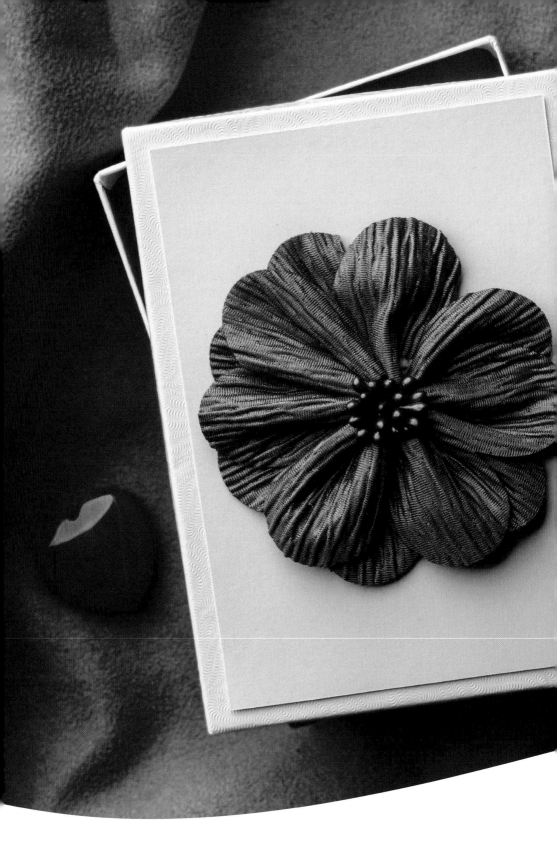

CHAPTER 17

Managing everyone else

I saw Rose for her postpartum visit after a late second trimester preg-nancy loss. She and her husband talked with their 4-year-old daugh-ter about how the baby wouldn't be coming home with them. Their daughter seemed to be handling the loss well. But Rose told me that while grocery shopping, her daughter ran up to a stranger and said, "Mommy had a baby in her belly, but it died."

The focus of this book so far has been on the person physically carrying the pregnancy. This is the person who must decide how to manage the miscarriage and the one who must deal with the physical process of losing the baby. But the loss im-pacts others in your life, including your partner, other children and extended family members. In this chapter, I talk about how everybody else might be experiencing what may feel like your private loss.

YOUR PARTNER

Even your partner, who may be your best friend, is reacting to a different experience than you are. Your partner, while not un-dergoing the miscarriage itself, is experiencing a loss, too.

Because the loss isn't physically happening to your partner, it may have a different psychological or emotional impact. I use the word *men* a lot in this section because the published research is limited almost exclusively to male partners.

Stereotypical behavior

Male partners may retreat into a stereotypical gender role, even if that's not their usual style or MO in a relationship. The expectation of the strong male is powerful in society, especially when his partner is vulnerable or sad. Some men have trouble expressing how they feel and may hold in their emotions — or even deny that they're having feelings at all.

We can't dismiss the pervasiveness of male bravado, and some men have a fear of losing face and need to maintain the facade that nothing is wrong for them. Many men do seem to cry less than many women and may feel less of a need to talk about a loss, even if you're desperate to talk about it with him. These reactions don't mean that he's not grieving, but for some men, trying to be strong means putting their feelings aside to be there for their partners. Your partner may struggle to express his feelings, holding in or denying his emotions in an attempt to be "strong" and support you the way he may feel like he should. This is especially true if he feels like the miscarriage threatens his masculinity, confidence or self-worth.

Uncertainty

For many men, watching their partners go through a miscarriage leads to a lot of conflict in which they don't know what to do for their partners or for themselves. This makes them feel utterly powerless. Many men feel very ill-prepared for what happens after a miscarriage. They're often placed in a support role by the medical team or by family or friends. Or they may volunteer for that role instead of focusing on their own grief. Research suggests that almost half of men whose partners miscarry never speak about their grief with their partners for fear of saying the wrong thing because they believe that the focus is supposed to be on their partners.

These feelings aren't entirely unfounded. Most of the support system around miscarriage — books, medical professionals or what little literature or pop culture references exist — is about how the person who has a miscarriage is coping with the loss. As a result, there's huge pressure for your partner to help you. Your grief is seen as more legitimate, and there are messages, both subtle and explicit, that your partner's grief will just add to yours. In some cases, men get the message that they're being selfish by thinking about their own feelings of loss.

Many men then feel that they need to recover quickly and are too busy coping with their partners' feelings to consider their own. These expectations around being a good partner and supporting you can lead to a huge Catch-22. If your partner openly shares his feelings with you to get the support he needs, he may only make your feelings worse because you'll feel concerned about him when you're going through a tremendous loss. But at the same time, if your partner doesn't show his feelings, he may come across as uncaring and unemotional, which also makes things worse for you. Caught between these two extremes, many men don't know how to respond.

Men may also feel uncertainty about what the miscarriage means for their *own* health. In the same way that getting pregnant and carrying a baby defines womanhood for some people, being able to get someone pregnant is associated with manhood and a sense of virility. Yet most of the focus is likely to remain on the pregnant person, both in managing the miscarriage and completing the medical work-up afterward. Few doctors will bring your male partner into the discussion until after multiple appointments with you.

Expressing feelings differently

Even when men do allow themselves to express their feelings about the miscarriage, this expression may look different from yours. Some men may mask their grief over the miscarriage with anger. Your partner may feel angry because he feels that the pregnancy's failure damages his image as someone who is healthy and potent. Or it may be because others don't recognize his very legitimate grief and confine him to this helper role as if he did not experience a loss as well. This anger may be directed at the doctors, himself or even at you.

I had a patient who brought her husband to her post-miscarriage appointment, and she said that they both felt that it must be her fault that the baby died. It became clear that her husband had placed the blame for the miscarriage on her, so I gently explained to both of them that no one was to blame (as I talked about in Chapter 1). Eventually, her husband got to a point where he could support her instead of blaming her.

Men may immerse themselves in work or other activities to avoid sharing their feelings or talking about the loss. Obviously though, some men may just not want to talk about it or to talk as much as their partners do. Some men don't want to be vulnerable in front of you or in front of family or friends. Some feel that people wouldn't understand their feelings. It can be hard to acknowledge their feelings even to themselves, and some may morosely wonder, "What's the point?" of talking about it because, "Talking about it won't change anything." This reticence to share their feelings may be the reason why some men may resist seeking professional help when grieving. It's less acceptable in many parts of society for men to seek help or therapy.

To show you a male partner's perspective, I asked my husband, Chad, to relive his feelings during and after our miscarriage. Even now, we have different perspectives about the day of the loss and the months after … but we agree that we handled the loss very differently. Read Chad's story on page 290.

Feelings of isolation

This idea that men need to be strong and shouldn't seek support from other people can then be compounded by a lack of volunteered support from friends, colleagues or family. Men don't frequently get asked as much about how they're doing with the loss. They don't get the support at work or from friends or family. This can make men feel isolated or on the outside of the miscarriage experience.

Some men feel like they don't know how to cope with the loss in an effective way. They're frustrated by the lack of information they're given about the loss. How often do your doctors talk to you, but not necessarily to your partner? He may be unable to explain the loss to other people or to himself and is left out of support systems that simply aren't built for partners.

Men often aren't treated as a patient or someone who's experienced a miscarriage in the health care system in the same way their partners are. They can feel excluded from what's happening. If your loss was particularly traumatic, involving hemorrhage, a trip to the hospital in an ambulance, a hospital stay or emergency surgery, there is also the trauma that they feel from watching someone they love go through such an event.

Bystander trauma — a consequence of watching someone you love be grievously injured and, in some cases, almost die — is not fully recognized or acknowledged nearly enough. Doctors and the health care system refer to the "second victims" of accidents, the circle of people connected to the person who was in the accident and how they're affected by the event. This is no different from what your partner may be going through based on your own traumatic miscarriage experience.

Wielding the Fire

By Chad S. White

When we lost our first baby at 7 months, Kate and I had dramatically different experiences. She was unconscious, having passed out from blood loss during an X-ray to try to diagnose what was wrong with her — whereas I got to watch as she became unresponsive, listen from the other side of the ER curtain as they cut her open and pulled out our lifeless daughter, and wait for hours as Kate underwent surgery to repair her exploded splenic artery.

It was 16 of the most anxious hours of my life. I don't enjoy thinking or talking about it because it was not only the day that we lost Samantha, but it was also the day that I almost lost Kate.

For me, the two are forever intertwined, but the latter was always more traumatic. When Kate finally woke up post-surgery, it was another anxiety-filled hour before she asked what happened to our baby. "She didn't make it," I said as I wept. "But we can make more babies. I only need you."

For months afterward, I worried that Kate had another aneurysm waiting to blow. When she would get caught in traffic from a Yankees game and be late coming home from work, I would have a horrible feeling that she was bleeding to death in her Civic on the Grand Central Parkway.

And for years, I was haunted by the sounds that Kate made when she became unresponsive during that X-ray. It was like the rhythmic whining of a faulty appliance, and in a noisy city like New York, I would regularly hear a sound on the street or in the subway that echoed it. I think that moving away from

New York City is one of the ways that I healed. Routine CT and MRI scans to confirm that she's free of other aneurysms also has helped.

Sometimes I feel bad that I wasn't able to better help Kate work through her grief. Early on, it probably seemed to Kate that I was trying to forget what happened or pretend that it never happened at all. Honestly, part of me wishes I could. But really, I just needed some time for the intensity of the fire to die down. I'm grateful to Kate's therapist, Andrea, for standing in the fire with her when I couldn't.

Now that time has passed, it's less painful. We recently celebrated our 15th wedding anniversary and we have two boys, 12 and 10. We'll never know, but I'm fairly certain that if Samantha had lived, we wouldn't have had our second son, Dexter, who is delightfully creative and affectionate. I can't imagine our lives without him, so I find comfort in that.

I also find comfort in writing, which is what I do for a living. It's therapeutic to apply my professional skills to what happened to us. I helped Kate write the opening of her article for *Glamour* magazine about her miscarriage, and I was an alpha reader and copy editor on this book. I'm also writing my first novel, a sci-fi epic about a girl, thought to have died at birth, who is reunited with her father just before her 18th birthday. Her name is Samantha, and she helps save the world.

It feels good to be able to wield the fire of our loss to make something positive, even if it does occasionally singe my sleeves. I hope that in time, you're able to handle your own fire and use it as a light to help others as well.

Deep grief

In the midst of all this discussion of how men may think about a miscarriage or how they choose to talk about it, it's important to know that most men feel deep grief about the loss. They may not show such intense personal despair, but that doesn't mean they don't feel it. One British study found that although men displayed fewer external signs of grief than their female partners did, they were more vulnerable to feelings of despair and difficulty coping in the first two months following the loss.

Everyone has limits beyond which they have trouble functioning or coping. Men may be overcome by the idea that they can't support their partners in the ways they need. In turn, they may feel that what they do isn't enough.

Pace of recovery

A difference in timelines for grief is a stressor that can affect how a couple deals with a miscarriage. Put simply, your grief timeline may be different from your partner's. Your partner may seem to move on more quickly than you do — partly because your partner wasn't the one who was pregnant, partly because it may be your partner's style of grieving. Your partner may not think about the miscarriage as time goes on and get concerned when you aren't recovering at the same pace.

Sadly, in some situations, people feel burdened by their partners' depression and irritation and by their "not getting over it." These conflicting reactions to loss and healing can be brutal on a relationship. I remember grieving in the months following my first loss and trying to talk with my husband, Chad, about my despair. He told me, "I don't want to be down where you are." It was hard for him to comfort me when doing so caused him enormous pain. I felt more alone than ever but tried not to blame him for not wanting to verbally process his grief. I recognized that it was just his way of coping. But feeling that your partner is moving on in some way without you may affect how you relate to him, as well as worsen your depression.

Impact on your relationship

Experiencing such a traumatic situation together may bring you closer at first. But grief, especially if you process the situation differently, can cause you to drift apart. Often, you may wonder why your partner doesn't seem more upset, and your partner may wonder why you're still struggling. Like me with my husband, you may need to talk it out, while he wants time alone. You may feel that there's no person in the world you want to process the loss with other than the person who's also experiencing it, but that person may feel like he just can't talk about it as much or as often as you want to. And of course, it could be the exact opposite, where your partner is still processing the loss and you're ready to move on.

These differing reactions about grief can upend your sex life. Sex can be genuinely life-affirming — a way to seek closeness and reaffirm your bond as a couple. But you and your partner may have different attitudes toward intimacy. One of you may be really missing the other physically and be desperate to be intimate again. And the other may have no desire for sex at all.

Sex and pregnancy are so closely intertwined for heterosexual couples that one of you may be reminded of the pregnancy by thoughts about sex. Additionally, either of you may feel vulnerable by the act of sex itself, thinking about its relationship to conception and to loss. And of course, the next pregnancy (whether you want it or not) hangs over the idea of resuming sex again. You may not be in the same mindset about trying again; one of you may be eager to get pregnant to put the miscarriage behind you, while the other needs more time to grieve. Read more about getting pregnant again in Chapter 19.

Same-sex couples

When it comes to same-sex couples, there is much less research compared with heterosexual partners, but pregnancy loss within lesbian relationships can be just as devastating. Non-pregnant partners can have the same response as heterosexual men do after a miscarriage, where they feel like they lose connection with their partners. Gay couples may find themselves in a similar situation when a surrogate carrying a pregnancy for them miscarries. Lesbian and gay couples may also face stressors from those in their lives and in society who don't support their becoming parents in the first place. Their grief may not be as socially acceptable — or even recognized.

Finding ways to connect

Everyone grieves differently. Just as you can't expect your partner to grieve the same way you do, your partner can't expect you to push your emotions aside and move on. It's important to be real about your loss, confront your grief and keep the lines of communication open with your partner. Above all, keep your common experience in mind: Giving up your expectations, hopes and dreams for a baby that won't be born is a major source of grief and pain for both of you.

Your partner needs you as much as you need your partner. If your partner is receptive, talk about what you're feeling. Is your partner feeling blamed, carrying guilt, feeling uncertain or feeling alone? The more that both of you can express your feelings — even if these expressions are different — the healthier you're both going to be in the long run, both as individuals and as a couple. The hard work comes from trying to understand your partner without judging him or her, even though that's so difficult to do. It's important to find common ground in talking about the loss that balances one person's need to talk about it and the other person's dread of talking about it.

I've heard therapists recommend a 20-minute rule for difficult conversations, when you literally set a timer and each person has 10 minutes to talk about whatever he or she is going through. It's a 10-minute space for you to be open about your feelings and for the other person to listen, and then the roles reverse and you listen to your partner. For some couples, when one person is desperate to avoid talking about the miscarriage, this might be a good compromise that creates a space to talk that's not open-ended.

In the same way, it's important to talk about how you're feeling about sex. Share your feelings and find a way to be intimate. You may need to consciously separate sex for fun and sex for function: The first is to enjoy being together, and the second is with the intention of becoming pregnant.

And don't forget that you don't have to have sex to connect. There are plenty of ways to be intimate together with or without orgasm that don't involve intercourse, which may be painful or scary for at least a little while.

CHILDREN AT HOME

If you have children at home, you'll have to find a way to talk about the pregnancy loss with them and help them cope with their feelings about your miscarriage. They'll need an explanation for why you had to go to the doctor or the hospital, or why you seem to be sad or mad all the time.

You don't have to hide your sadness from your children. (Trust me, they're going to pick up on it anyway.) Trying to hide your feelings compounds their uncertainty and confusion about what's happening. Let yourself cry in front of your children to let them know that expressing sadness together is OK. Similarly, sharing your feelings with them about the baby or about the pregnancy with them gives them a safe space to talk about their feelings in return. And it lets your kids know that all feelings are OK. Even if you haven't had the kind of household or relationship with your kids where you've talked about feelings much, this is a critical time to convey that feelings are natural and need to be expressed in a healthy and safe way.

Let people who watch your kiddos — a babysitter, the child care center workers, a nanny — know about the situation. Talk to them about how your children are taking the news and perhaps what they've been doing or saying in response. You can even let caregivers know how you'd like them to answer any questions about the pregnancy loss and if there are any things that you don't want them to talk about.

Children may have mixed emotions about the loss, no matter their age. Kids may simply be sad about the loss of a sibling. They may feel guilty if they were harboring any feelings of resentment about your being pregnant. Children may be angry that they did not get the sibling they were hoping for or were promised. Or kids may not even react at all, especially if they're young. For some children, the concept of miscarriage is too abstract to understand, or too scary to discuss.

All of these feelings — including having all of them at once — are completely natural for children in the same way it's understandable for you and your partner to feel conflicted. So it's important to respect their reactions and not pressure them to talk about what's happening if they don't want to.

Going forward after the loss, you may want your children to participate in rituals or ceremonies that you plan. Whether they do depends on your kiddos, what they're expressing and their emotional maturity. Don't force your children to take part in a funeral or other ceremony if they're not ready to do so.

If you were hospitalized or you had multiple doctor's office visits because of your miscarriage, your children's typical routines may have been disrupted — maybe a lot. As soon as you're able to, restore your kids' routines for meals, school, activities and sleep. Even in the worst of circumstances, children thrive under routines. Restoring routines sends the message that life is continuing as it was for them, even if that's not exactly what you're feeling inside. If you made any promises to your child about what would happen after the baby came, like a big-kid bed or a different room, follow through if it's at all possible. Otherwise, it may cause resentment and stir up negative feelings and emotions.

Once you're ready, spend special time with your kids to remind them that they're safe and show them how much you love them. Children may interpret your sadness as rejection, so show them how important they are to you. Caring for your kids may make your grief easier. There's something about taking a break from focusing on your own pain and focusing on the needs of others for a while that eases grief a little bit. It can also remind you that you're already a parent and that having a child can happen for you again.

Paradoxically though, caring for your children can make it harder for you to heal. You may feel sad when caring for your older children when thinking about caring for the newborn that you expected to have. Your kids don't really have anyone to talk to except for you and your partner, so you're going to bear the brunt of their feelings, their questions and their processing, which can be exhausting. If you'd rather stay in bed than make lunches, bring the kids to school, give them baths or help with homework, then running headlong into parenting as you're physically and emotionally healing can be tough.

Accept help for taking care of your kids at this time, whether it means splitting tasks with your partner or getting help from others who might volunteer to take the kids for a while to give you some space. Both you and your kids need time to process the loss of pregnancy.

I can validate that having kids and going through a miscarriage can make it both better and worse, and that your feelings are legitimate. Do what you need to assist your own healing and be the great parent to your kids that you always are.

Young children

Young children — in the pre-tween years — mostly want to know two things: Are they still safe and loved, and is their parent going to be OK? Your children may be feeling a variety of things about the baby, but you're their parent and you're their world. It's OK to tell children that you're sad about the baby and to say that you may be hurting a bit.

For the youngest kiddos, you may want to say that you've been sick and a nice doctor at the hospital is making you feel better, but you're still sad to feel so sick. I tend to use "sick" a lot with my own kids as a synonym for sadness, anxiety, stress — you name it. If your kids knew you were pregnant, explain that the baby wasn't growing properly or that it couldn't stay inside you any longer.

This may be your children's first exposure to death, which can make this conversation more difficult. Now is the time to explain that everything that lives at some point dies. You can talk about how death brings room for new life, but this may be too vague when talking about the new life that is a pregnancy. The U.K.-based Miscarriage Association has multiple suggestions for how parents can talk to very young children. (Learn more in the Resources section of this book.) One idea is to compare pregnancy to planting seeds in a garden and explain that only some seeds grow into full plants. Preschoolers may think that death is reversible or temporary, so you may need to repeat your explanations about death before they understand. Keep your information straight and simple, without too many details, and avoid such words as "sleep" or "went away," as these may sow confusion (or terror) the next time they go to bed or are left with a sitter. It's not until they reach school age that children start to understand what death is, but they may believe that it can be avoided or won't affect them. If your family is religious or spiritual, you may be able to use tenets of your faith to talk about the loss.

Children's emotions often come out in their behaviors, like bedwetting, night terrors, and hyperactivity or inappropriate laughing. Giggling, for example, might represent not joy but expressions of anxiety — especially when children are hearing talk about the pregnancy or the baby. Kids may shift shockingly quickly between feeling sad and feeling happy, and their behavior doesn't always match their underlying emotion.

Older children

Give your tweens and teens a high-level view of what happened — that you were pregnant, but the baby wasn't healthy and died, and you needed to see a doctor (and perhaps have a procedure) to make sure you were OK. You can focus on the fact that you're safe now but still feeling sad that there won't be a new baby in the family.

Talk about the loss in simple but truthful ways, and let your children's questions guide you. Children will ask what they're ready to know; you don't need to give them answers to questions they're not asking. For instance, when I was talking to my husband about this book over dinner one night, my then-10- and 8-year-old boys asked what it was about. When I said it was about miscarriages and explained what those were, my youngest reacted by saying, "Thank goodness that never happened to us." When I told him that it had, in fact, happened to me, his eyes widened. But rather than asking any questions at all, he simply hugged me — and then went back to eating his chicken nuggets. (I'm always amazed at the resiliency of kids.)

If they do have questions, they may ask about you, how you're doing and how your body is doing. They may want to know why miscarriage or stillbirth happens. And questions may also be about themselves, about what the miscarriage means for them, about not being able to hold or play with the baby or do other things that now won't happen.

It's important to reassure your kids that the loss had nothing to do with them. Make sure they know any bad feelings or thoughts they had did not make the miscarriage happen, even if they felt jealous about a new sibling. While some kids may express jealousy to you, other kids will hide it in shame or fear. Call it out and let them know that it's completely OK. It's important for children to know that nothing could have been done to prevent the miscarriage. And you can even let them know that if part of them is relieved that there won't be a new baby taking all their parents' attention, that doesn't make them bad people.

It's not uncommon for children to react in inappropriate or regressive ways, like having outbursts at siblings or classmates, or to have their performance in school dip. Talk to your children's teachers about what's happening at home and ask for understanding, especially if you see it impacting your children's behavior or performance at school.

FAMILY AND FRIENDS

Just when you've told everyone in your house and you're all grieving together, you now remember that there are people outside your doors who care about your well-being and knew about the pregnancy and now need to know that it's over.

Your family and friends bring their own history of pregnancy or miscarriage to your situation. Many people can check this at the door and just be there for you in the ways that you need them to be. Others may be so upset for you that you may end up comforting *them*. I lost track of how many people stopped me at work to cry on my shoulder — in the hallways, in the elevators, in the *bathroom*. Each time I hugged them and patted them on the back, a small voice in my head was screaming, *Are you kidding me?!*

Family and friends may not realize just how upset you are, especially as time goes on. Way too quickly, it will feel that they start treating you as if the pregnancy loss didn't happen. They may not realize that you want to talk about the loss even weeks or months later. Conversely, your family and friends may bring up the loss a lot and ask you how you're doing, how you're feeling and what your plans are when you would rather grieve in private and don't want to talk about it with them or in wider circles.

Help them help you. Your family and friends love you — even if they don't always know what to do or say — and genuinely want to comfort you. Let them know whether you want to talk or just need their support doing anything else but talking. Remember, no one can read your mind. If you decide to talk with people, let them know how you want them to react. Do you just want them to listen and to comfort you, or do you want them to actively help you process? This is an issue that I've had with my analytical, problem-solving husband. When I just want Chad to listen and acknowledge my feelings, I simply tell him so — otherwise I know I'm going to get cool-headed (but loving) strategizing.

People very often say, "If there's anything I can do … " which they genuinely mean, but it's not often helpful. When people say this to you, give them things to do, whether it's grocery shopping, housecleaning, helping with your kids or driving you to doctor's appointments. People are often thrilled to be able to help you in your time of need. But if you're not specific, you may end up with 15 casseroles stacked up in your freezer.

(No judgments if that's what you'd prefer.) Take a look at the letter at the end of this chapter for ideas on how to communicate your needs to others.

Another task to ask for help with is spreading the word about your miscarriage among your extended social network. You shouldn't feel the need to tell the whole world that you lost your pregnancy — even a couple of phone calls may be agonizing — so it's reasonable to ask a few friends and family members to spread the word to your larger circle so that you don't have to tell everyone. Not every cousin or work associate needs to get a personal phone call from you about your loss. Delegate that to your closest aunt or best friend at work.

Allow yourself to feel your feelings. You don't have to be strong for others. You are the one who experienced a loss. It's OK to not be strong and to expect others to be strong for you.

WHO HAD THE LOSS?

All of our parents expressed sadness after our pregnancy losses. Our first loss, a daughter early in the third trimester, devastated my mother-in-law, who desperately wanted a girl in the family after raising my husband and his brother. During every visit and every phone call, she would bring the conversation back to our loss. But she always framed it as *her* loss. We felt like we comforted her more than she comforted us and that it was her feelings and hopes and dreams we discussed more than our own. It was so much that Chad eventually told her outright to stop talking about the baby in front of us. We had our own grief to manage and simply could not take on hers as well.

Co-workers

How soon you return to work depends on your physical health and how many vacation or sick days you have. I have some patients who go back to work three days after a dilation and curettage (D&C). Others can take a month or two off after a stillbirth. If your miscarriage is an ectopic or a molar pregnancy that requires multiple trips to a lab for blood draws, you may still be actively managing your miscarriage while at work.

Your doctor can give you a note for work or school that explains that you're receiving care, especially on multiple days. The note can specify when you're medically cleared to go back to work but can withhold details. Not everyone feels comfortable sharing a personal situation at work or school.

If your company doesn't include miscarriage as a reason to take paid maternity leave, you may qualify for up to 12 weeks of unpaid leave from work through the Family and Medical Leave Act. There are detailed questions to determine if you're eligible, about the size of the company and how many hours you've worked in the past year. Talk to your human resources department or get more information in the Resources section of this book. Unpaid leave may not be feasible for you and your family, but it's good to know it's an option.

Work may distract you from your grief. It can be therapeutic to throw yourself into a task that has nothing to do with your pregnancy. Work can remind you of the things you enjoy in life, and you may have friends at work who don't remind you of the loss. And if you drive to work, you may find that being alone in your car provides a space for emotional breakdowns when you need them. It may be a relief to get out of your house, especially if you have reminders of your pregnancy at home.

On the other hand, work may be incredibly difficult once you're back on-site. You may find it tough to concentrate or

PREGNANT WHILE TRANS

People of all genders can and do become pregnant. Transgender men — those who identify as men but were assigned female sex at birth — commonly use the hormone testosterone as part of their medical transition. Ovulation usually stops within 6 to 12 months of starting testosterone, but trans men retain their egg reserves, and ovulation may intermittently occur after that. It's very possible to become pregnant in the first year of testosterone therapy without contraception, and less likely but possible after.

The idea of transgender men becoming pregnant may strike some as strange, as pregnancy is so strongly associated with being female. Yet it's completely understandable for any person to want to become a parent, including having a genetic link to a child. After all, no one asks cisgender folks why *they* want to have a biological child. In studies, transgender people give the same reasons that cis people do for wanting to have children, including connection with their partners and wanting to form a larger family.

All people who hope to become pregnant need prenatal counseling that includes both routine topics like prenatal vitamins and genetic screening and a review of medications, including testosterone, and when to stop taking them before conceiving. While pre-pregnancy use of testosterone doesn't appear to affect the health of the baby or the pregnancy, exposure to testosterone during pregnancy can cause birth defects. Other than that, the medical and obstetric care for transgender men is the same as that for any pregnancy. Recommendations for prenatal diagnosis options, lab testing, ultrasounds and fetal surveillance are the same for all pregnant people.

It's no easy decision to stop gender-affirming hormonal therapy. Some transgender men experience worsening distress from the difference between their gender identity and their sex assigned at birth (gender dysphoria), depression, and a deep sense of isolation. Even if they were planning to become pregnant, the pregnancy itself can feel foreign and alienating. But for most transgender men, being pregnant is a wonderful bonding experience with their babies, just like it is for cis women.

We know the language and context around pregnancy and birth is highly gendered — women's health, maternity ward. This lack of inclusion of those with diverse gender identities can make it hard to seek care, and trans people often delay or don't seek it, or align with nontraditional health care providers. Once they do present for care, transgender men may face uncomfortable or unwilling providers, improper care, wrong advice, and misgendering by staff. And if they are not out as trans, they may have even more challenges.

All of this means that having a miscarriage can be even more emotionally devastating for someone who is transgender. While the topics discussed throughout the book apply to all pregnant people, transgender men must also wrestle with lack of acceptance of their pregnancies and the feeling of a different kind of betrayal by their bodies.

Make sure you reach out to the people in your life who will support you through this time and through your journey toward parenthood. And don't hesitate to switch health care providers if your team isn't providing you with the information you need and the support you deserve.

you may be easily distracted. For a while, work may just not feel that important compared with the loss. Be kind to yourself, and don't expect things to feel normal right away.

You may have lost your pregnancy early enough that many colleagues didn't know you were pregnant. In this scenario, you may want to continue to separate your work life from your personal experience of loss, especially if you don't feel close to any of your co-workers. The saving grace of no one knowing at work is that no one will ask you questions or bring up the pregnancy unexpectedly. They may also unintentionally say or do things that trigger your sadness. The downside is that colleagues may unintentionally say or do things that trigger your sadness. If they don't know about your loss, they can't offer you support, but this may be less important if your social network is outside of your workplace.

If you had a miscarriage after co-workers knew you were pregnant, on the other hand, you'll have to decide how you want to share the news of your loss. Some colleagues may know about the loss, but there will likely be some who haven't heard what happened. As I mentioned earlier, consider delegating the task of sharing the news of your miscarriage to a trusted friend at work, or possibly a human resources manager depending on the size of your company. Especially if you experienced a stillbirth or had started to arrange maternity leave, you don't want to go back to questions from all sides about what happened. And if you've had a baby shower? I'm sure people will understand if you're not up to sending thank-you cards.

My first miscarriage happened in a dramatic way while I was at work. I collapsed while giving a lecture and was brought by ambulance to the emergency room. By the time I returned to the office after my recovery, my entire department knew the details. It was a relief to have people know, but it required a lot of, "I'm fine, thank you, it's OK," when my co-workers came up to me and wanted to talk about what happened. I'm a fairly touchy person, but even I became hugged-out by the number of comforting embraces I was offered. I found myself saying I was fine a lot, even when I wasn't, because it was the quickest way to exit the conversation. One thing I didn't expect was how many people would then tell me their own stories of loss or those of a close friend or sister. These conversations were meant to be helpful — misery loves company, I'm not alone, yadda, yadda, yadda — but it's rough to have to listen to everyone else's horror when you're dealing with your own. I was even trapped in an elevator once, for 16 floors, with someone who kept expressing sympathy and trying to get me to talk about how I was doing.

I understood that all these folks meant well and were trying to relate, but each talk opened the wound, and I felt so drained by it. I was at work, the one place where I didn't want to break down and cry, especially anywhere near my boss. I felt less alone by knowing how many people cared and hearing how many people had losses of their own. But it was a struggle to manage everyone else's feelings along with my own. And for months I would occasionally run into far-flung work acquaintances who congratulated me on the baby with a cheer. *Those* were awkward conversations.

My advice for people whose colleagues know about their pregnancy loss is to set boundaries for yourself. It's OK to only want to talk about your grief with a few close work friends, and not want to rehash what happened or how you're feeling with every single person. And you don't have to talk about it at work at all if you don't want to. Let everyone know — through an email or through a friend — that you appreciate the warm wishes, but you want to focus on your job without thinking about the miscarriage (at least when you don't want to). My husband emailed his boss to tell her what happened and asked her to relay the news to everyone, as well as let them all know that he didn't want to talk about it. He was greeted with greetings of welcome back but no unwelcome questions.

GET WHAT YOU NEED FROM YOUR SUPPORT NETWORK

Dear _____ ,

You're receiving this letter because you're someone who cares about me. I'm having a hard time with my pregnancy loss, and I know you want to help me. So if you are looking for specific ways to help, I would really welcome:

☐ Flowers and cards

☐ Food baskets

☐ Prepared or freezer-friendly meals

☐ Grocery shopping

☐ Child care

☐ Help with housework

☐ Help with yardwork

☐ Rides to doctor's appointments

☐ _____

☐ _____

Even more than tasks and things, it's important to me that my family and friends acknowledge the baby and the loss rather than avoid the topic. Give me space to talk, to be open and to grieve. Let me weep without jumping in to comfort me – right now, your presence and your love is all the comfort you can give me. Don't tell me it's going to be OK, because right now, it's not OK.

What to say to me:

☐ I'm sorry.

☐ What can I do to help?

☐ Would you like to talk?

☐ I'm here to listen.

☐ I don't know what to say, but I love you.

☐ _____

☐ _____

What **not** to say to me:

☐ Anything that starts with "At least" including:

    o   At least you know you can get pregnant.

    o   At least it was early in the pregnancy.

    o   At least you didn't really know the baby.

☐ You can try again/you'll get pregnant again/you're young.

☐ You already have one child (you should be grateful)/ you can always adopt.

☐ This is God's plan for you/it was God's will.

☐ Time heals all wounds.

☐ Everything happens for a reason/it happened for the best/it wasn't meant to be.

☐ You're stressing too much.

☐ Thank goodness you have your health.

☐ There was something wrong with the baby anyway.

☐ It's not like losing a child who has lived with you.

☐ I know exactly how you feel.

☐ _____

☐ _____

Thank you for everything—your support means the world to me.

HOW TO ASK FOR SUPPORT

Something I have heard from many patients is that they don't want to talk to friends or family about their loss. And the most common reason is because they don't want to feel like a burden on the people they love. It breaks my heart to see patients turn away potential sources of caring and support because they're thinking about the needs of their networks before their own needs.

Perhaps every friend or family member may not be able to help you in the same way, especially if they're facing a crisis of their own at the same time. But if someone you loved was hurting, wouldn't you want to be able to help them if you could?

Please don't think of reaching out for support as burdening your family and friends. Helping one another is part of what makes a family and a community. So let yours help you when you're needing their love the most.

Every family recovering from a loss needs something different — and everyone receives a different level of support from his or her network. If you're like me, you may find it difficult (or maybe even excruciating) to ask for what you need.

So in the spirit of "what I wish I had when I had a miscarriage," I've created a guide you can copy and give to people who are persistently asking what they can do — and to people who have foot-in-mouth syndrome and are constantly saying the wrong thing. You'll find it on pages 308 and 309.

Check the boxes for the things you need and use the open lines to write in others. Or visit *www.drkatewhite.com* to download an editable version that you can email to your support network.

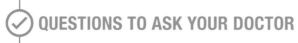

⊘ QUESTIONS TO ASK YOUR DOCTOR

Bring this list of questions to ask your doctor about helping the others in your life manage their grief and about how to help them help you. Take notes and check off the questions as you go.

☐ Do you know of local support groups or services that my partner can use?

_____

☐ Do you have any resources for how I can talk to my children about the miscarriage?

_____

☐ How can I tell if my kids are doing OK?

_____

☐ Can you give me a letter for work that explains what happened so I don't have to talk about it?

_____

☐ Do you know of resources or therapists who are experienced in working with gay, lesbian or trans clients?

_____

_____

_____

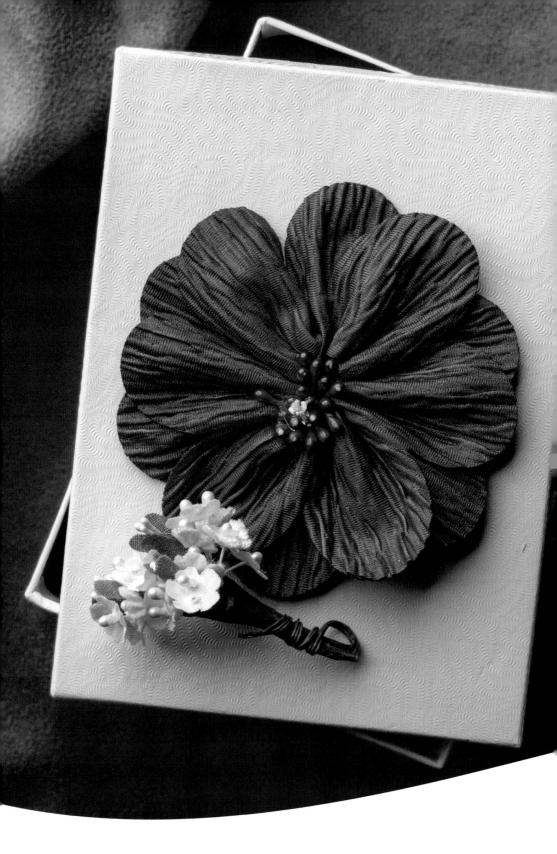

CHAPTER 18

Ways to remember

Sarai, a mother of three, found herself unexpectedly and happily pregnant with her fourth baby. So she was devastated the day that the doctor told her that there was no heartbeat on the ultrasound. She was 5 months along when she chose a surgical procedure.

Afterward, in recovery, we were able to give her the baby to hold and say goodbye to. As Sarai held her daughter, tears fell from her face to the baby's face. She told me she planned to tattoo the baby's name on her back, right below the names of her other children.

One of the reasons that I think people feel so unmoored after a miscarriage is that the U.S. lacks cultural traditions around mourning and remembering babies lost through miscarriage. Because you're grieving the potential that this baby held and the hopes and dreams that you had for his or her future — rather than grieving the time that you spent with the child — it's seen as less deserving of the comforting memorial and funeral rituals that surround other deaths.

This reflects part of the bias around the way in which a pregnancy is lost. Parents who experience a stillbirth can access the full spectrum of bereavement services: They can see a spiritual adviser, get a funeral home referral, and have conversations about burial or cremation. And people who experience a second trimester fetal death may be offered some of these things. Research shows that parents offered such ritual intervention are much more satisfied with their care.

But with a first trimester pregnancy loss, it's not common for a medical care team to bring up bereavement options. And many medical care providers don't even see an ectopic pregnancy as a miscarriage. They focus on the medical intervention to save the parent's life and often don't spend much, if any, time on the pregnancy that was lost. And most people aren't given leave from work to recover after a miscarriage. They have to choose between vacation time or unpaid leave.

Partially because of this lack of traditions and ritual around early pregnancy loss, and partially due to the insensitivity of the medical community, people who experience pregnancy loss and their families must create their own paths through grief and remembrance. For some people, this is a critical step that they need to take before they can fully heal and move forward in a healthy way. What follows in this chapter are examples of what people have done to memorialize a miscarriage.

That said, you're not expected to do any of these things. Nor should you plan a funeral, name your baby or do anything else you don't want to. Many families don't feel the need for formal ceremonies or remembrances, and that's fine. It's up to you and your family to decide what feels right to you, on the timeline that feels right to you. Even if a lot of time has passed since your pregnancy loss, it's never too late to remember that pregnancy in a special way.

The gestational age at which a pregnancy ended isn't a reason to do or not do any of these things. It's only about how you want to process the loss and to what degree you want this remembrance to be a part of your life.

AFTER AN INDUCTION

After going through labor in the second or third trimester of pregnancy, you have the opportunity to see your baby after delivery. Many people find that having an opportunity to hold the baby briefly and say goodbye provides true closure to a pregnancy, especially one in which they felt the baby moving inside of them.

Not all people are offered this opportunity after delivery. Some providers think that you will be too tired or too sad to hold the baby. But if this is something that is important to you, do not hesitate to speak up ahead of the procedure. This is your child after all, and you should have a chance to say goodbye.

You may also have the chance to bathe and clothe the baby, if you wish, or to have a religious ceremony like a baptism with a pastor from the hospital or your own. Some families want to take pictures of the baby. You may do this yourself or use a hospital photographer. If you're not sure if you want to take a picture home at this point, your doctor can likely put it in your medical chart in case you want to retrieve it later. You can often have footprints of the baby made or save locks of the baby's hair if the pregnancy was very advanced.

Many hospitals will offer you a memory box to be able to keep things from the pregnancy, blankets that wrapped the baby in the hospital, ultrasound pictures, or a certificate of life, which is an unofficial birth certificate that marks the occurrence of your baby's birth. You can also place in this box photos of you while you were pregnant, any special items that you made or bought for your baby, or other items sent to you for your pregnancy or for your loss, such as cards, small gifts or dried flowers. If you're not offered a memory box, ask for one. My box from my first loss holds a small album of ultrasound pictures, my hospital bracelet, a card with the baby's footprints and the overalls that I bought for her the day I learned I was pregnant.

MEMORY BOXES

Memory boxes and what you put inside allow you to memorialize your pregnancy in a way that brings you comfort.

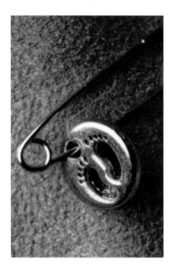

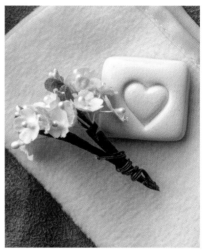

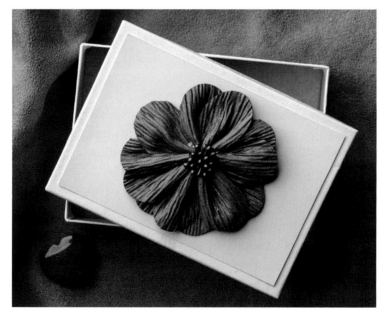

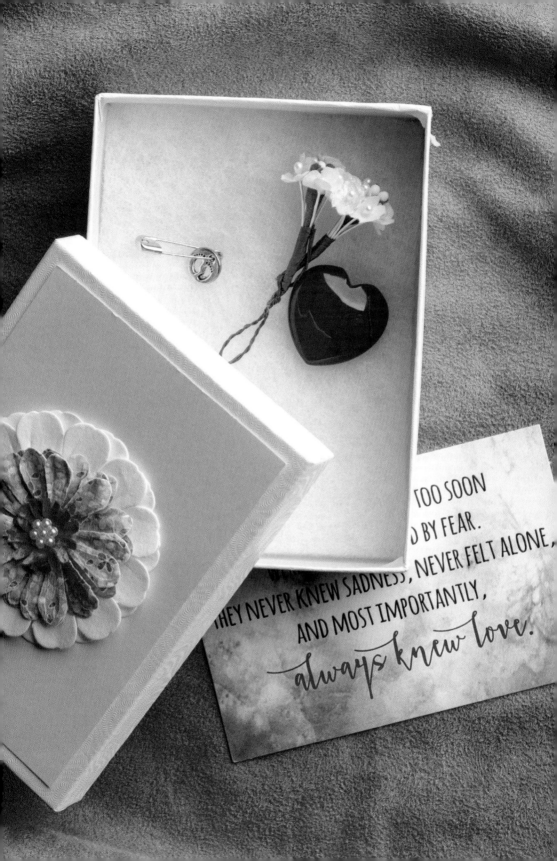

AFTER AN EARLY LOSS

With a loss in the first trimester of pregnancy, you may not be offered the same types of keepsakes. However, you can still request a memory box — ask the providers to get you one from labor and delivery if they're not sure what to do when you ask.

If they don't have memory boxes, you can make your own. Craft and hobby stores offer wooden boxes of all shapes and sizes. You can decorate them or leave them unadorned. If you're crafty, you can create a needlepoint box with plastic canvas squares. The size of the box depends on what you want to put inside. Any small box can hold ultrasound pictures, a certificate of life, a pregnancy test or lab results, or anything small you purchased for the baby, like socks or a onesie. I make memory boxes for my patients to add to (see pages 316 and 317). They contain silk forget-me-not flowers, a tiny footprint pin or charm, and a heart-shaped stone. Put anything in your box that has meaning for you so you can memorialize your pregnancy in a way that brings you comfort.

Patients have told me that they like to have something in their pocket that they can reach in and touch if they're thinking about the baby and they want such a moment to be private. So while some people are comfortable wearing a necklace that refers to the baby or the pregnancy, others want something more hidden. Something like a memory stone can be great for this purpose. The hearts photographed throughout this book are just this type of keepsake. They're from Grief Watch, which is listed in the Resources section.

NAMING THE BABY

While cultural and religious traditions vary on this subject, for my patients, naming the baby makes the baby real to them. Giving your child a name recognizes this baby as a part of your

WHAT TO PUT IN YOUR MEMORY BOX

The possibilities are endless, but here are some items to consider:

Tokens from the pregnancy
- Your positive pregnancy test
- Photos of you during your pregnancy
- Ultrasound photos
- Photos of the baby taken after delivery
- Your hospital ID bracelet or your baby's
- A certificate of life from the hospital (you may need to ask for this)

Items of remembrance
- Silk forget-me-not flowers
- A footprint pin or charm
- A memory stone

Gifts to the baby
- Cards you received
- A tiny handmade blanket
- Jewelry

Gifts from you
- A letter you wrote to the baby
- A special outfit, socks or shoes
- A poem that you've written, or one of your favorites

family. This baby left a mark on your life and your family. Naming the baby may be a way to honor that. For our daughter, we had talked the most about the name Samantha. While we hadn't decided on a name before her delivery, once I held her, it was clear that Samantha was her name after all.

MARKING THE MOMENT

Some people like to do something in private once they've found out they've had a miscarriage or shortly after they've passed the pregnancy.

For example, you may write a letter to your baby about how you felt when you got pregnant, what being pregnant was like, or the dreams and wishes you had for your baby's future. Sometimes, writing these thoughts down gives you a concrete way to say goodbye. You can save this letter in your memory box, you can bury it, or you can burn it and scatter the ashes in a body of water or in a meaningful place. If you're a digital person at heart, consider creating a Pinterest board to pin images and quotations and other things that make you think about the pregnancy in a healing way.

CEREMONIES

Some people find comfort in traditional religious services with clergy, family and close friends. Both religious and cultural traditions can provide memorial services and other ceremonies, like Christian baptism, that help remember lost pregnancies.

Nonreligious memorials are often referred to as remembrance ceremonies. These include a ritual and a time to think about what the pregnancy meant to you. This can be a ceremony that you have with family and friends or it can be as simple as just you and your partner, or even you alone.

As part of your ceremony, you may do something like:
- Go to the beach when the tide is going out and set flowers, driftwood or pine cones in the water.
- Scatter seeds in the wind in a place where they can grow.
- Read a poem or recite song lyrics that are meaningful to you or the pregnancy.

CUSTOMS FOR PREGNANCY LOSS AROUND THE WORLD

In my research for this book, I came across rituals from around the world created to help families grieve pregnancy losses. In addition to the rituals and traditions of your own culture or religion, you may be inspired by some of these:

- In Mexico, Indonesia, Japan, South Africa and New Zealand, families create variations of symbolic "surrogate baby" dolls to represent the lost baby.
- In southern Ghana, women mourning a miscarriages might enter the forest, bathe in a river, make offerings to appease their gods, and then be painted with white clay and dressed in white cloth.
- In Japan, the practice of *mizuko kuyō* (meaning water child memorial service) begins with crafting a cap, bib or necklace. A ceremony may include words to Jizō, the guardian of the souls of *mizuko*, a word that refers to stillborn, miscarried or aborted fetuses. A statue of Jizō may be placed on the grounds of the temple or at home after the ceremony. These rituals may be offered at Zen centers in the U.S. In Taiwan, a similar practice known as *yingling gongyang*, is observed.

- Plant a tree in your garden or local park or arboretum. My husband and I planted a tree in our backyard in remembrance of our daughter in each house we have lived in since the loss.
- Send compostable balloons into the air, maybe with a message inside of one or writing on them.
- Bury a note along with flowers or mementos.

After any of these acts, you can follow with a short prayer, meditation or just quiet reflection.

BURIAL

Whether or not you decide to bury your baby depends on your family. Hospital staff often ask about burial for second or third trimester losses or stillbirths but will rarely ask about it for first trimester losses.

If your hospital asks if you're interested in burial, it is by no means an indicator that you should be. While some families want to have funeral ceremonies and burial services, many families don't need any kind of burial for healing. So please do not feel obligated.

Some hospitals offer burial of the baby at the hospital's expense in a local cemetery. Very often, multiple pregnancies are interred all together in a special area of the cemetery, so no markers are placed for your baby alone.

If you decide to proceed with a private burial, you will be advised to communicate with a funeral home while you're still in the hospital or shortly after you leave. The funeral home arranges to transfer the baby from the hospital after testing. You won't be given the baby yourself to take out of the hospital, but instead the transfer will go through the funeral home the same way it would for the burial of anyone else.

Many funeral homes offer remembrance packages for families that have lost a pregnancy or newborn. It's typically inexpensive — even free in some cases. So while the wild cost of funerals is well known, don't let anticipated high costs deter you from a burial for your miscarriage if it's something you want.

Depending on your local funeral homes and cemeteries, you may have the option to have a marker placed where your baby is buried. Sometimes you can have a marker placed even without a burial of the baby. Talk to the funeral director to get information about your options.

If burial or cremation is important to you, *tell your doctor that you're interested in this option as soon as possible*, because the paperwork gets filed very differently when the baby is to be held for burial. If you aren't sure if private burial or cremation is right for you but you think it might be, tell your doctor this, too. The hospital will err on the side of keeping the baby and giving you time to make this decision. Once you decide on hospital disposition of the baby, there's no way to change course, so if any part of you thinks that you want a private service, let your doctor know.

DONATIONS IN YOUR BABY'S MEMORY

If a donation is within your means, choose a charity that seems meaningful or appropriate to you to donate in your baby's memory. You can donate any items or clothing that you may have received as gifts or bought for the baby to a hospital, women's shelter or other such charities. You can donate toys, books or money in your baby's name to a local children's hospital or library, favorite charity, or school. You can make a memorial donation to a pregnancy loss support group. You can even endow a scholarship in your baby's name, perhaps at a local school or one that means something to your family, or for students pursuing a career in health care or a field that has significance for your family.

When I told the story of my first pregnancy loss in *Glamour*, I donated payment for the article to the March of Dimes, which does amazing work in pregnancy loss prevention. For me, that seemed like the perfect way to remember my daughter.

ONGOING PERSONAL REMEMBRANCES

You may find that the annual recurrence of a meaningful date becomes a focal point for a remembrance ritual. Your ritual may be something that you want to do on that particular day, or it may become an ongoing symbol of the baby.

Ways to remember the anniversary of your loss or when the baby was due may include:

- Planting perennial or annual flowers in your own garden or in a community garden.
- Selecting an item to keep as a visual remembrance of your baby. This could be a stuffed animal, a small statue of the baby or of a mother and child, a music box, or a Christmas ornament. My husband, Chad, named a star after our daughter. He also bought a special star-shaped Christmas tree topper in her honor. In these ways, our daughter is a part of all our holiday celebrations.
- Wearing a piece of jewelry for your child — a ring, charm on a bracelet, or locket on a necklace — that's inscribed with your baby's name or has a birthstone for when your baby was due.
- Writing a letter to your baby every year on the anniversary of the loss or due date and keeping the letters in your memory box. The first letter could be about how you felt when you found out you were pregnant, your hopes and dreams for the baby's future, and what the miscarriage meant to you and your family. Future letters could be about your feelings about the future, your family, or simply how much you miss your baby. Since I have lousy handwriting (typical doctor), I've typed multiple letters to my daughter, emailed them to myself and saved them in a private folder.
- Writing poetry to your baby to express the feelings you never got to say to him or her.
- Making a cross-stitch or creating a needlepoint with your child's name and remembrance date and turning it into a wall hanging or pillow.
- Lighting a candle and having either a private or a family ceremony.
- Sending flowers to a hospital to be given to any mom who's experiencing a loss.

- Creating a quilt to hang, use or donate.
- Donating blood every year on the day of the miscarriage. This very physical act helps other people, possibly even those who are pregnant.
- Sending baked goods or other food or supplies to a support group for bereaved parents that might have helped you in the first year after your loss.

The bottom line is to do what feels right for you and your family. Ceremonies and traditions can help you manage the short-term shock and grief of a loss and help shape your grief into easier ways to remember over time. Simple or complicated, religious or secular, the point of all these remembrances is to help bring the grief out of the dark, make it public, validate it and share it with those you love so that it doesn't haunt you.

Pain is intensified when it's private and hidden, so consider these kinds of remembrances or any of your own as a way of marking this important part of your journey in your life.

✓ SELF-REFLECTION AFTER A LOSS

You might not be ready to think about how to memorialize your pregnancy for many days, weeks or even months after your loss. As time passes, you may want to reflect on what steps you can take to remember your pregnancy. Use these questions to help guide you.

☐ Do you have any family customs about how to remember a person who has died?

_____

_____

_____

☐ Would you like to draw on religious or cultural traditions or rituals?

_____

_____

_____

☐ If you haven't talked with your partner about how to remember the pregnancy, do you want to begin that conversation?

_____

_____

☐ Who do you want to include in your thinking about ceremonies or actions to remember the baby — your partner?
Your family? Your other children?

_____

_____

_____

_____

☐ Put a star next to the ideas in this chapter that speak to
you. Which ones do you think you want to consider for
making your own remembrances?

_____

_____

_____

_____

☐ If it's been a long time since your loss, do you think you
would like to remember your pregnancy in one of these
ways?

_____

_____

_____

PART 5

Moving forward

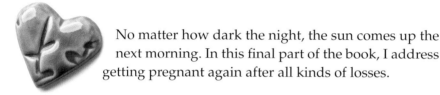

No matter how dark the night, the sun comes up the next morning. In this final part of the book, I address getting pregnant again after all kinds of losses.

I also share with you my personal story of loss and discuss how we're all part of a larger community that can give us strength, courage and hope for what's to come.

CHAPTER 19

Getting pregnant again

Thea saw me two months after her miscarriage. She was healing well and back at work. I asked her about what her thoughts were about getting pregnant again. Sighing, Thea told me that her husband was very anxious about trying again for a baby. "But I don't know, I'm less sure," she said. "I'm so afraid of having another miscarriage. I don't know if I can go through that again."

Some people want to fully grieve their pregnancy loss before even thinking about getting pregnant again, and some people feel that the best way to heal after a loss is another pregnancy. Those in the latter group often think, *Well, if I want to be a parent, the best way to get over being sad about not being a parent is to try again.* There is no right or wrong answer as to when you should try — if ever — to get pregnant again after a miscarriage. In this chapter, I discuss the decision-making around when to try to conceive again after a miscarriage.

FIRST TRIMESTER MISCARRIAGE

The long-standing advice from doctors used to be to wait 3 to 6 months after a miscarriage before trying to get pregnant again. The thinking was that you wanted to have several regular cycles of your period after the loss to make sure everything had returned to the way it was before you tried again. But studies have now shown that there is no benefit to such a wait.

For my patients, I advise that they wait until their first regular period after the loss before trying to conceive. Knowing the date of your last menstrual period lets you and your doctor know how far along you should be in the early weeks. Waiting this long allows doctors to have a more accurate dating of the next pregnancy (instead of guessing when you got pregnant).

But there's no medically proven reason to wait even that long. There's no apparent impact on the health of the next pregnancy if you get pregnant sooner or later after a miscarriage. Besides the advantage of getting a clear estimation of the date of your next pregnancy, there's no reason you can't start trying to get pregnant again right away after a first trimester loss.

SECOND TRIMESTER LOSS

In general, you don't need to wait to become pregnant again after a pregnancy loss in the second trimester. Whether you had a dilation and evacuation (D&E) or a labor induction, I advise waiting only until your two-week follow-up visit, just to make sure there were no complications with regard to bleeding or infection. But that's it in terms of waiting.

The other element for some people is that they might want to wait for the results of testing that was done on the pregnancy tissue if their doctor thinks that these tests will reveal a condition that needs attention before the next pregnancy.

Talk to your doctor. If the reason for the loss is clear, or there's no reason to wait for testing, you can try to conceive as soon as you want to.

THIRD TRIMESTER LOSS

For stillbirths in the third trimester, it can get a little more complicated. If you had a labor induction, delivered the baby without complications and have no trauma to your vagina, there's no reason to wait to have sex again.

But as for getting pregnant again, you'll want to talk with your doctor. Some studies say it's safe to try again for pregnancy as soon as you want to. But other studies say you may be at risk of pregnancy complications if you conceive in the 18 months following a stillbirth.

It's possible that you'll be able to get pregnant again as soon as three or four weeks after the pregnancy loss. So you'll want to decide with your partner if it's more important to you to get pregnant as soon as you can, or if you want to delay to reduce any possible risks to you or the next baby. Additionally, you may want to wait for the results of medical testing on you or the baby if you think it may reveal something you might want to consider before trying to get pregnant again.

If you needed a C-section, which is uncommon, the best way to go is to let the incision on your uterus heal first. You want the surgical incision on your uterus to transform into a firm, healthy scar before a new pregnancy causes the uterine muscle to stretch and expand against the scar. In this case, it's healthier to wait at least six months, if not a year, before trying to conceive. It may sound horrible to have to wait that long, but after a C-section for a pregnancy loss in the third trimester, your body needs time to heal before it's safe to try again.

Ectopic pregnancy

Ectopic pregnancies are a special kind of miscarriage, and they're also different in terms of timing for trying to conceive again. If your ectopic pregnancy was treated medically with methotrexate injections, the drug must clear your body before you become pregnant again. Because there's no definitive evidence that it is safe to get pregnant again soon after taking methotrexate, many doctors advise waiting a few months. You also want to wait for your pregnancy hormone level to reach zero to confirm that the pregnancy is truly over.

If your ectopic pregnancy was treated surgically, the usual advice after a laparoscopy is to wait 2 to 3 weeks to have sex so your scars have time to heal. But there's no evidence for that, either. You probably don't want to have vigorous, athletic intercourse a few days after surgery (not that most people are in the mood for that anyway), but there's no real good estimate for how long you should wait to have sex after an uncomplicated surgery. While waiting two weeks is probably a safe bet, I'm not sure that you need to wait six weeks. If you're unsure about how long to wait after an ectopic pregnancy loss, talk with your doctor about what makes the most sense for you.

Bottom line: Listen to your body. If sex hurts — in your belly or in your pelvis or elsewhere — don't do it. That's pretty good advice for life in general.

As for the rare kinds of ectopic pregnancies — those in the cervix, or in a C-section scar or in the horn (cornua) of the uterus — the general advice is to wait six months before becoming pregnant again. These tissues are less equipped to handle a pregnancy, so they need plenty of time to heal before the uterus is home to another growing pregnancy.

MOLAR PREGNANCY

This is the hardest one of all. As you learned in Chapter 11, before getting pregnant again, you must wait until your human chorionic gonadotropin (HCG) hormone levels reach zero and stay there for six months to a year. That's because if you get pregnant while your doctor is monitoring your hormone levels, the doctor won't know if a positive pregnancy test and rise in HCG levels is a new pregnancy or the now-cancerous tissue of the previous molar pregnancy. In that case, you wouldn't know if you are pregnant ... or need chemotherapy.

This is one kind of pregnancy loss where all the advice is clear: You need to wait for the all-clear from your doctor before you try to conceive again.

TERMINATION FOR MATERNAL HEALTH OR FETAL REASONS

If you were in the first trimester, you'll be able to try for pregnancy again as soon as you feel ready. After a surgical procedure, your doctor will let you know if there's any reason you should delay trying. If you used medication, you'll likely have a follow-up ultrasound to confirm passage of all the pregnancy tissue. Once you know the pregnancy is truly over, you can try to get pregnant again.

If your termination was in the second trimester, it's a similar situation. You'll likely have a follow-up visit to make sure your body is healing, whether you had a surgical procedure or a labor induction. After that, you're good to go.

In both situations, your fertility is going to return within weeks of your loss. So if you want to delay your next conception, talk with your doctor about your birth control options.

CHANCES OF ANOTHER PREGNANCY

In terms of what your chances are of pregnancy after a pregnancy loss, they're pretty much the same as before, based on

TIMES YOU NEED TO DELAY PREGNANCY

For some kinds of pregnancy loss, you need to work with your doctor to determine the right timeline for trying to get pregnant again. In these cases, it can be months or even a year after your loss before it's safe to start trying again.

- **Stillbirth with a cesarean section.** The scar on your uterus needs to fully heal before the uterine muscle can safely stretch to accommodate a new pregnancy.
- **Ectopic pregnancy treated with medication.** You'll need to monitor your blood pregnancy hormone levels until they have reached zero to make sure there is no remaining pregnancy tissue before a new pregnancy begins. You also want to make sure all of the methotrexate medication leaves your system so it doesn't harm your next pregnancy.
- **Cornual, cervical or scar ectopic pregnancy.** When a pregnancy sac implants in an unusual part of your uterus, your body needs more time to heal before it's safe to conceive again.
- **Molar pregnancy.** Doctors are only sure that all the pregnancy tissue has left your body once the pregnancy hormone levels have reached zero. And if you have had a complete molar pregnancy, the recommendation is to wait 6 to 12 months to ensure that the pregnancy tissue has not turned cancerous and started growing again.

your age, health, and fertility. Once you feel that you've healed enough — body and soul — from your miscarriage to consider getting pregnant again and your doctor has given you the all-clear, you can start thinking about what timing is best for you and your family to try to be pregnant. As you look ahead toward trying again, here are ways to address some of the common concerns you may have at this point.

Genetic counseling

Genetic abnormalities are the most common reason for losses in the first trimester, which is the reason why doctors don't tend to perform genetic testing for first trimester miscarriages. For most people, the genetic abnormalities don't repeat, so while you may have an answer to *why*, it doesn't really help you the next time around.

If you've had multiple losses with your partner, or your second or third trimester miscarriage was caused by a genetic condition, you should consider seeing a genetic counselor. These counselors help you understand how genetic conditions and birth defects run in families and can help you figure out the chances of this condition recurring.

The wonderful thing about these visits is that the counselors can take a long time to sit with you, go over your family tree, and hear about other people in the family who might have been affected by this illness or condition. They can spend time with you to talk through the implications, what testing would be recommended for you and what it means for getting pregnant in the future. Counselors overall spend a lot more time with you than a doctor can, so while your doctor may know some of this information, I still recommend sitting down with a genetic counselor to get the best kind of counseling possible. Your doctor's office can help you figure out if a genetic consultation would be covered by your insurance.

Chances of another miscarriage

Many of my patients, like Thea, worry about their miscarriage risk with another pregnancy. Happily, with a first trimester loss, the most common kind of miscarriage, the odds are that your next pregnancy will be healthy. As scary as the miscarriage was, the odds are very much in your favor of having a healthy baby the next time out. And first trimester miscarriages that weren't ectopic pregnancies do not make you "high risk" in your next pregnancy. However, do keep an eye out for cramps or bleeding and tell your doctor if you notice anything.

With a second trimester loss, the chance of another miscarriage depends somewhat on the reason for the first loss. Many of the reasons why people lose a pregnancy in the middle are reasons that don't repeat. This goes for third trimester stillbirth, too. About 1% to 3% of women who had a stillbirth have another stillbirth, so while there is an increased risk of another pregnancy loss with these later losses, the vast majority of women will go on to have a healthy baby with their next pregnancy.

If you've had a pregnancy loss in the second or third trimester, you'll likely be considered higher risk in your next pregnancy. Your doctor's office will likely stress the importance of keeping your prenatal appointments and all appointments for all your testing. For most people, it doesn't require a visit to a high-risk obstetric specialist or a maternal-fetal medicine (MFM) doctor. However, if a complicated medical condition led to your pregnancy loss, your doctor may feel more comfortable if you see an MFM specialist in the next pregnancy.

MFM doctors have years of specialized training in taking care of pregnant people with conditions that require management or monitoring during pregnancy. If you have complex diabetes, antiphospholipid antibody syndrome or another condition that may complicate your pregnancy, you may be safer seeing an MFM specialist if one is available to you in your area.

After you've had an ectopic pregnancy, you are at an increased risk of having another one. After one ectopic pregnancy, you have a 10% risk of having another one — and this risk goes up to 25% after you've had two or more ectopic pregnancies. As scary as these numbers may sound, it still means that 75% to 90% of the time, your next pregnancy will be in the right place.

If you've had an ectopic pregnancy in the past, your doctor will monitor you closely with an early ultrasound.

With a molar pregnancy, your risk of recurrence is much lower, between 1% and 9%. This number is closer to 1% to 2% in the U.S. From an optimistic point of view, this means 91% to 99% of pregnancies that follow are healthy. With a history of a molar pregnancy, you'll get an ultrasound early in the first trimester to confirm that everything looks healthy.

PREVENTING ANOTHER LOSS

Almost all my patients ask me what they can do to prevent another miscarriage. There are very, *very* few reasons that a first trimester miscarriage occurs that can be addressed in a follow-up pregnancy. Throughout the book, you've learned about the risk factors for pregnancy loss — such as age, race and family history — and most of them can't be changed.

But there are a few things you *can* do to improve your chances of preventing a miscarriage:
- Avoid alcohol, tobacco, vaping, marijuana and other non-prescribed substances before and during pregnancy.
- Work with your doctor to maximize your health before and during pregnancy, including switching your medications to those that are safe for pregnancy.

That's it. Unfortunately, there are only so many things you can control when it comes to the first trimester of pregnancy. The best thing you can do is to accept that you have so little control.

My patients who've experienced a second or third trimester loss are anxious about such a loss happening again. Many causes of stillbirth are, sadly, unknown or unpredictable. The things that you can do are the things that any person should do to lower the risk of losing a pregnancy in the third trimester.

IF THIS WAS YOUR FINAL PREGNANCY

I wrote this book to not only to give a deeper understanding of pregnancy loss, but also to provide hope for future attempts at pregnancy. But I know that for some people reading this book, their pregnancy loss was their last chance. Perhaps you've been through "too many" miscarriages, and you or your partner can't emotionally attempt another pregnancy. Perhaps you had a medical condition that has led your doctors to tell you that becoming pregnant again would be life-threatening. Or perhaps you transplanted your last frozen embryo and you're not able to try in vitro fertilization (IVF) again. Many of you may have been on your pregnancy journey for a long time and find that the road just … ends.

Accepting that you're not going to be able to have a (or another) pregnancy may feel like a part of you has died. Your grief is valid. It hurts on the very deepest level to not be able to have the family that you may have pictured for a long time, and the loss of this dream compounds the loss of your pregnancy.

When you're ready, you can think about what comes next for you. It may be pursuing adoption or leaning into being an aunt or uncle. Maybe you will find joy volunteering with youth in your community or finding other ways to help kiddos in need. And you may go in an entirely different direction — embracing the particular freedoms that come with not having young children to care for, or finding new ways to have joy with the family that you've already created.

For now, though, allow yourself the space and time to mourn all that you've lost. Surround yourself with people who can support you. And know that there are other satisfying roads ahead for you to travel.

1: Have a preconception visit with your doctor to make sure that you're as healthy as can be before getting pregnant again. This is the way to make sure that you're managing any medical conditions with as few medications as possible, and that you're on medications that are safe for a pregnancy.

2: Get as close to a healthy weight as possible before getting pregnant. There's evidence that being overweight is linked to a higher risk of stillbirth. There's nothing easy about losing weight after a pregnancy. It's even harder than trying to lose weight at other times. If this is one of your goals, consider seeing a nutritionist or a weight-loss specialist who can help.

3: Quit smoking tobacco and marijuana, and don't use alcohol or other nonprescription drugs.

Once you're pregnant again, it's important to seek out prenatal care early and to make sure your doctor knows that you have a history of stillbirth. You'll want to be alert during this pregnancy for anything unusual, like cramping or pain or any bleeding from your vagina. And once your pregnancy is far enough along, your doctor will teach you how to do kick counts, which are a way for you to monitor the baby's well-being every day.

PREGNANCY AND MENTAL HEALTH

Some people think that getting pregnant again is the best way to get over grief, that anxiety and depression symptoms will go away once you give birth to a healthy baby. Unfortunately, simply having another pregnancy doesn't end grief or protect against these symptoms. Research shows that women who've had miscarriages are at greater risk of depression and anxiety in their next pregnancies. Even if you're thrilled beyond belief to be pregnant again, prolonged or complicated grief after a loss puts you at risk of prenatal or postpartum depression.

This is a good reminder that depression is *not* the same as sadness. You can be incredibly happy about being pregnant and still be at risk. That's because depression is a neurochemical imbalance that has nothing to do with your mood, gratitude or self-worth. I would say the most high-risk part of your next pregnancy isn't the miscarriage itself but the depression you may have gone through while you were healing.

---

⑦ YOU MAY BE THINKING ...

I'm pregnant again, but I'm so afraid to tell anyone yet because I'm afraid of another miscarriage.

First, congratulations! And second, it's perfectly understandable to want to keep the pregnancy a secret for a while. Do what feels right to you. If there are people in your life who you know would be supportive and who you feel comfortable talking to, you might consider telling those people, even at this point, even before the first trimester screening. Let them share in your joy, because they'll be the ones to share in your sorrow if lightning were to strike again.

Pregnancies are practically snowflakes. If you ask someone who has multiple children, or even multiple pregnancies, they often state that each pregnancy was very unlike the one before. Whether it's nausea, energy levels or cravings, every pregnancy is a discrete event. You get to reset the clock and start down a new, hopeful road. Having a pregnancy loss in your past, while always having a place in your heart and your medical record, doesn't affect the baby to come. If you are able to, you should enjoy this next pregnancy and all the possibilities that it holds.

The risk of depression starts as early as when you become pregnant and lasts through the first year after your baby's birth. The first few weeks postpartum, for example, can be difficult if you've had a pregnancy loss in the past. You may have conflicted feelings about all the joy surrounding this baby, comparing it to the pregnancy you lost before. You may feel the stark difference between the support that you're now getting with an infant at home compared with the silence or discomfort of others at the time of your miscarriage.

These feelings are normal. Talk about them with people you love or a therapist, if need be, so that you don't feel guilt or shame for very natural reactions after a pregnancy loss. Your doctor will likely ask if your grief persisted for more than a couple of months after your miscarriage. Your doctor can also look out for signs of perinatal depression, which can be treated with counseling and medication, even during pregnancy.

Warning signs to watch for

If you're experiencing any of these warning signs, consider talking with your doctor or midwife:
- Feelings of sadness that affect your daily functioning at home, with your family, at school or at work
- Difficulty sleeping in the first or second trimester (it's common to have disrupted sleep in the third trimester)
- Obsessing about the current pregnancy
- Going to the doctor repeatedly and requesting test after test

LOOKING AHEAD (AND BEHIND)

Even amid the joy of having a newborn, it can be important to take a moment to reflect on and remember the pregnancy that you lost that you wanted just as much. The birth of a baby may offer an opportunity to reflect on the pregnancy you lost and acknowledge that joy and sadness can be felt at the same time. It's not disrespectful to the pregnancy you lost to find delight in giving birth to or adopting a baby. You can both remember the pain of the past pregnancy, and look ahead to the future with hope for this new little one.

The birth of a new child may be a good time to think about the remembrance rituals in Chapter 18. If you haven't yet done something specific to mark your previous pregnancy or incorporate the memory of your miscarriage into holiday or annual occasions, you may want to consider doing this now. It may be less painful, in fact, to think about the pregnancy you lost now that you've been able to bring a baby home.

When my beloved editor at *Glamour* asked me about writing the story of my pregnancy loss for the magazine, I told her, "Not until I have my happy ending." I needed to be able to

---

(?) YOU MAY BE THINKING …

I'm excited to be pregnant again, but I'm also scared.

It's completely normal to feel scared during your next pregnancy, especially up until the point at which you lost the last pregnancy. If you had a miscarriage at eight weeks, you might hold your breath until you reach nine weeks. If you lost your baby at seven months, you may feel better once you make it to eight months. Some people won't relax until they are holding that baby in the delivery room.

Share these feelings with your partner or your closest supporters. If the fear threatens to overwhelm your joy and the experience of being pregnant again, consider talking to a therapist who can help you manage these feelings.

give birth to a baby who lived before I could consider writing about the one who didn't. Two years later, once I held Zachary in my arms in the recovery room after my semi-urgent cesarean section, I knew that I was ready to share my story.

✓ QUESTIONS TO ASK YOUR DOCTOR

Bring this list of questions to your appointment to ask regarding your options for trying to conceive after miscarriage. Take notes and check off the questions as you go.

☐ When is it safe for me to start trying for pregnancy?

_____

☐ Is there anything I should do for my health before getting pregnant again?

_____

☐ Do you think it would be good for me to see a genetic counselor before I get pregnant?

_____

☐ Should I be worried about depression in my next pregnancy?

_____

☐ If I don't get pregnant in the next six months, what can I do?

_____

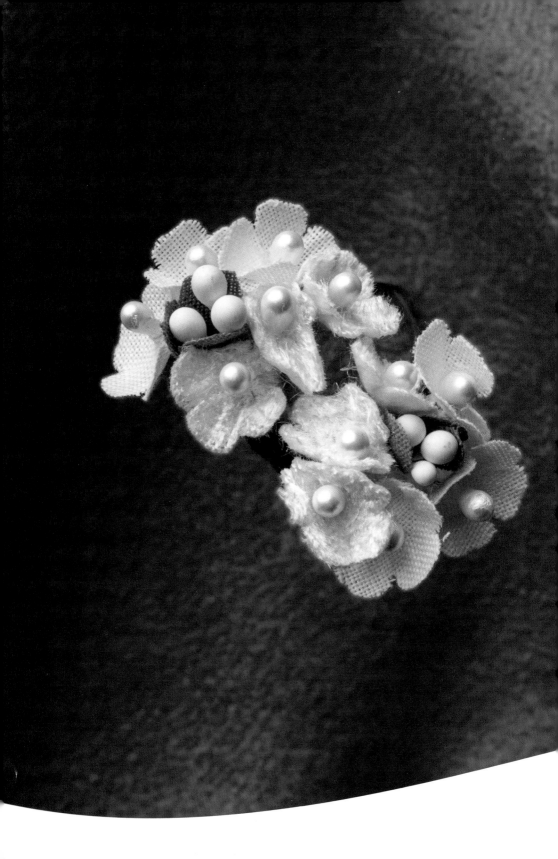

CHAPTER 20

Final thoughts

Kate, a 35-year-old pregnant doctor, collapsed while giving a lecture to residents at her hospital. She was rushed to the labor and delivery unit, but her doctors couldn't tell what was wrong with her. When the baby's heart rate on the monitor started to dip, the doctors almost performed an emergency C-section. However, they decided to wait because she was only 7 months along. When she later became unconscious during an X-ray to try to diagnose the problem, they went ahead with the emergency cesarean, but the baby had already died. It turns out that an aneurysm on Kate's splenic artery had ruptured. She lost her baby, her spleen and most of her blood volume that day — and nearly her life. When she woke up the next morning, she had no memory of what had happened.

At the start of the book, I said that a miscarriage could truly happen to anyone. That's because when I was 35, it happened to me. For the longest time, I felt completely broken. I had wanted to be a mother more than anything, and I felt like my body had betrayed me in the deepest way possible.

I did not know how I was going to continue, especially being a doctor who took care of pregnant people every single day. I found myself managing everyone else's pain around the loss

— friends, co-workers and family members. Hospital co-workers would stop me in the hallway and start crying after hearing my story — and I found myself hugging them, telling them it was OK. All the while, a little voice in my head was whispering, *It's not OK!*

Once it was time to start trying to conceive again, my husband and I discovered that I needed assistance from a fertility specialist. I then experienced that combination of fear and anxiety. *What if I couldn't get pregnant again?* I asked myself over and over. *What if I never get to become a mother?* When I became pregnant again, I was so afraid of what would happen, both to me and to the pregnancy, that I didn't feel safe until I held the first of my two sons in my arms nine very long months later.

REDUCING THE STIGMA

Even though it's a common experience and nothing to be ashamed of, miscarriage has rarely been discussed in public. The undeserved stigma surrounding miscarriage has done real harm to the people who've experienced a loss, making them feel isolated, alone and guilty when they shouldn't.

Thankfully, in recent years, many people have stepped forward to tell their stories, including Chrissy Teigen and John Legend, Michelle Obama, Meghan Markle, Pink, Gwyneth Paltrow, Nicole Kidman, Halsey, Mariah Carey, Beyoncé, and Wendy Williams. In addition to those, other amazing, brave people have talked about their experience with multiple miscarriages, including Gabrielle Union, Courteney Cox, Celine Dion, Jaime King, Lily Allen, Priscilla Chan and Mark Zuckerberg, Kimberly and James Van der Beek, and Tana and Gordon Ramsay. Pregnancy loss doesn't discriminate.

With both my professional and my personal experience, I can tell you how common it is to feel so alone and so heartbroken after the loss of a pregnancy that you dearly want. Doctors treat miscarriages as routine, which is meant to be reassuring, but it's anything but routine for most people.

Society needs a better culture for how to handle pregnancy loss. We need to end the silence around miscarriage. Doctors and medical staff need to support people and their whole families when they're experiencing the loss of a pregnancy. We need to acknowledge their loss, grief and devastation. And we need to acknowledge that there's no one right way to talk about it or to experience it. A miscarriage can mean different things to different people. Some people may see it as a relief or a blessing, right alongside any grief they feel.

I used to routinely tell my pregnant patients that they shouldn't tell the world that they're pregnant until they're out of the first trimester. I thought there was too high a risk of miscarriage for patients to be open with their whole networks about a pregnancy that might well end in pregnancy loss.

But my thinking has evolved.

It's important for people to talk about their pregnancies early on so that if a miscarriage does happen, they'll know that they have other people they can talk with about it. I know that means putting yourself out there, which can be a little risky. But it's a far bigger risk to stay quiet and then experience a miscarriage and be alone.

If more of us can be open, then we create a world in which more people are able to talk about their experience of miscarriage in a supportive environment, and where their feelings of grief and loss are not only acknowledged and understood but also validated by their friends and family and the wider community. Friends and family of people experiencing pregnancy loss won't be afraid to ask them how they're coping, and those grieving miscarriage will feel comforted and supported by telling the truth. All these steps can reduce the stigma that's still associated with miscarriage.

I hope that sharing my own story has helped you in some small way. I hope that this book has made you feel less alone, and that it has helped you understand your situation and your options. Every day, I try to teach the next generation of doctors how to help people experiencing miscarriage and treat them with greater empathy and understanding.

You can help reduce the stigma around miscarriages, too. Can you join a support group? Can you reach out to a friend or co-worker who has experienced a miscarriage and be a source of support? Speak out as much as you're able about the loss. Help to demystify this for others.

You can even help improve the medical care that other people receive during their miscarriages. It may sound strange, but doctors can be just as awkward and ill at ease as other people in your life, and they don't always know how to support you. Through my own losses, I've found that doctors are more comfortable focusing on the medicine than on the emotions around miscarriage. So you may need to be proactive.

Ask your doctor and your medical team questions when they come up in your mind, or have your support person ask the questions for you. There's nothing you can't ask when it comes to you and your baby. If you want to see the pregnancy sac after a D&C, just ask. If you're concerned that your feelings of grief are unusual, just ask. If you don't know how to support your partner, just ask. When you're upfront about the help you need, your doctors can become more aware of the information they should routinely be giving to their patients.

Understand that your care must be individualized and that every person needs something different from doctors, partners and social networks. You're not asking for too much when you have a lot of questions. You're not indecisive when you want time to decide what to do. You're not needy when you want a follow-up visit to help process the loss. You're not complaining when you need to talk out your feelings about what has happened to you. And you're not weak when you recognize that you aren't coping well and need help. All these things make you smart, thoughtful, wise, open and brave.

You're entitled to feel the way that you do and to get what you need to feel better. Take as much time as you need for self-care around the miscarriage and don't let anyone convince you that your miscarriage is *just* anything — that it's *just* an early loss, *just* one loss, *just* not the right time, *just* not meant to be. Right now, it's your whole world, and that's OK.

Take as much time as you need when thinking about the next pregnancy, too. If thoughts about the next pregnancy give you comfort, then try to become pregnant again as soon as you can. But if you need more time to mourn this loss, take that time.

Hanging in my office at work is a quote that brings me comfort. The phrase seems to have originated with the Brazilian author Fernando Sabino, and then been popularized by John Lennon:

Everything will be OK in the end. If it's not OK, it's not the end.

I know from all the patients I've taken care of how strong and resilient people are, even when they feel like they're not going to survive the day. And from my own experience, I know that you can surround yourself with people who love you, who will genuinely help if you tell them what you need. I know that with the right medical team and the right care, you will heal from this loss. You will be OK.

Resources

I hope this book served as a guide through miscarriage, whether this was your first loss or you've had several miscarriages. Many organizations are devoted to providing resources for families experiencing pregnancy loss. Whether you prefer to read a book or surf the internet, information is available for you. You can also visit my website, *www.drkatewhite.com*, for a list of resources. Updates are made to it on an ongoing basis.

WEBSITES AND ORGANIZATIONS

American College of Obstetricians and Gynecologists
www.acog.org/womens-health/faqs/early-pregnancy-loss

American Pregnancy Association
https://americanpregnancy.org/getting-pregnant/pregnancy-complications/pregnancy-loss

American Psychological Association
www.apa.org/monitor/2012/06/miscarriage

American Society for Reproductive Medicine
www.reproductivefacts.org/topics/topics-index/miscarriage-or-recurrent-pregnancy-loss
www.reproductivefacts.org/topics/topics-index/ectopic-pregnancy

Baby Loss Family Advisors Baby Loss Doulas
www.babylossfamilyadvisors.org

Babyloss (UK)
www.babyloss.com

Centering and Grief Digest Magazine
http://centering.org

The Compassionate Friends
www.compassionatefriends.org

Depression Screening Tool
www.hiv.uw.edu/page/mental-health-screening/phq-2

Family and Medical Leave (FMLA)
www.dol.gov/general/topic/benefits-leave/fmla

Generalized Anxiety Disorder 2-item (GAD-2)
www.hiv.uw.edu/page/mental-health-screening/gad-2

Grief Watch
https://griefwatch.com/

A Heartbreaking Choice
www.aheartbreakingchoice.com

March of Dimes
www.marchofdimes.org/complications/loss-and-grief.aspx

Miscarriage Association (UK)
www.miscarriageassociation.org.uk

Miscarriage Support (New Zealand)
www.miscarriagesupport.org.nz

MISS Foundation
www.missfoundation.org

National Human Genome Research Institute
www.genome.gov/about-genomics/fact-sheets/chromosome-abnormalities-fact-sheet

National Organization for Rare Disorders
http://rarediseases.org/for-patients-and-families/information-resources/rare-disease-information

Now I Lay Me Down To Sleep
www.nilmdts.org

Postpartum Support International
www.postpartum.net

Seattle Children's Hospital
www.seattlechildrens.org/clinics/grief-and-loss

Share Pregnancy & Infant Loss Support Inc.
https://nationalshare.org

Star Legacy Foundation
https://starlegacyfoundation.org

Unspoken Grief
https://unspokengrief.com

Verywell Family
www.verywellfamily.com/miscarriage-support-organizations-2371339

BOOKS

Empty Arms: Hope and Support for Those Who Have Suffered a Miscarriage, Stillbirth, or Tubal Pregnancy
Vredevelt P. 2nd ed. Multnomah Publishers; 2001.

Empty Cradle, Broken Heart: Surviving the Death of Your Baby
Davis DL. Fulcrum Publishing; 2016.

An Exact Replica of a Figment of My Imagination: A Memoir
McCracken E. Little, Brown and Company; 2008.

Holiday Hope: Remembering Loved Ones During Special Times of the Year
Fairview Press. Fairview Press; 1998.

I Had a Miscarriage: A Memoir, A Movement
Zucker J. Feminist Press; 2021.

Knocked Up, Knocked Down: Postcards of Miscarriage and Other Misadventures From the Brink of Parenthood
Lemoine MM. Catalyst Book Press; 2010.

Life Touches Life: A Mother's Story of Stillbirth and Healing
Ash L. NewSage Press; 2004.

Not Broken: An Approachable Guide to Miscarriage and
Recurrent Pregnancy Loss
Shahine L. Lora Shahine; 2017.

Our Stories of Miscarriage: Healing With Words
Faldet R, et al., eds. Fairview Press; 1997.

The Prenatal Bombshell: Help and Hope When Continuing or
Ending a Precious Pregnancy After an Abnormal Diagnosis
Azri S, et al. Rowman & Littlefield; 2015.

The Rules Do Not Apply: A Memoir
Levy A. Random House; 2017.

A Silent Sorrow: Pregnancy Loss – Guidance and Support for
You and Your Family
Kohn I, et al. 2nd ed. Routledge; 2000.

Tears of Sorrow, Seeds of Hope: A Jewish Spiritual Companion
for Infertility and Pregnancy Loss
Cardin NB. 2nd ed. Jewish Lights Publishing; 2007.

They Were Still Born: Personal Stories About Stillbirth
Atlas JC, ed. Rowman & Littlefield; 2010.

Trying Again: A Guide to Pregnancy After Miscarriage,
Stillbirth, and Infant Loss
Douglas A, et al. Taylor Trade Publishing; 2000.

We're Going To Need More Wine
Union G. HarperCollins Publishers; 2017.

When a Baby Dies: A Handbook for Healing and Helping
Limbo RK, et al. Bereavement Services; 1986.

ARTICLES

7 Women on What a Miscarriage Feels Like
The Cut
www.thecut.com/article/7-women-on-what-a-miscarriage-feels-like.html

64 of the Best Things Ever Said to a Griever
What's Your Grief?
http://whatsyourgrief.com/what-should-i-say-to-someone-grieving

Are Men Forgotten in Miscarriage?
BBC News
www.bbc.com/news/health-41525610

Do Men Grieve Over a Miscarriage?
Parent24
www.parent24.com/Fertility/Miscarriage/do-men-grieve-over-a-miscarriage-20180214

The History of Talking About Miscarriage
The Cut
www.thecut.com/2018/04/the-history-of-talking-about-miscarriage.html

How a Man Handles a Miscarriage
The Art of Manliness
www.artofmanliness.com/articles/how-a-man-handles-a-miscarriage

Recognizing Miscarriage as an Occasion for Grief
The New York Times
www.nytimes.com/2020/10/19/well/family/pregnancy-loss-miscarriage.html (subscription required)

You Know Someone Who's Had a Miscarriage
The New York Times
www.nytimes.com/interactive/2019/10/10/opinion/miscarriage-pregnancy.html (subscription required)

RESOURCES ABOUT REMEMBERING

12 Rituals of Miscarriage
Fertility Resilience
http://fertilityresilience.com/12-rituals-of-miscarriage

Adopting a Buddhist Ritual to Mourn Miscarriage, Abortion
National Public Radio
www.npr.org/2015/08/15/429761386/adopting-a-buddhist-ritual-to-mourn-miscarriage-abortion

The Japanese Art of Grieving a Miscarriage
The New York Times
www.nytimes.com/2017/01/06/well/family/the-japanese-art-of-grieving-a-miscarriage.html (subscription required)

Pregnancy Loss
RitualWell
www.ritualwell.org/pregnancy-loss

Rituals
Empty Arms Bereavement Support
www.emptyarmsbereavement.org/rituals

TALKING TO CHILDREN ABOUT LOSS

Be Honest and Concrete: Tips for Talking to Kids About Death
National Public Radio
www.npr.org/2019/04/24/716702066/death-talking-with-kids-about-the-end

How to Talk to Your Child About Pregnancy Loss
BabyCenter
www.babycenter.com/pregnancy/your-life/how-to-talk-to-your-child-about-pregnancy-loss_10310179

How to Talk to Children About Miscarriage and Stillbirth
What's Your Grief?
http://www.whatsyourgrief.com/how-to-talk-to-children-about-miscarriage-stillbirth

Talking to Children About Miscarriage
Miscarriage Association
www.miscarriageassociation.org.uk/wp-content/uploads/2016/10/Talking-to-Children.pdf

Talking to Children About Miscarriage
Verywell Family
www.verywellfamily.com/talking-children-about-miscarriage-2371334

CHILDREN'S BOOKS ABOUT MISCARRIAGE

Molly's Rosebush
Cohn J. A. Whitman; 1994.

We Were Gonna Have a Baby, But We Had an Angel Instead
Schwiebert P. 5th ed. Grief Watch; 2018.

When Someone Very Special Dies: Children Can Learn to Cope With Grief
Heegaard M. Woodland Press; 1996.

Glossary

3D ultrasound. Like a regular ultrasound in that it uses sound waves to create a picture of the uterus. The extra dimension allows doctors to see if there are any abnormalities inside the uterine cavity that may be causing miscarriages.

acute stress disorder. Directly associated with a traumatic event. Can include a sense of numbness or lack of emotional responsiveness; feeling dazed or outside of oneself; reliving the event through recurrent thoughts, dreams or flashbacks; avoiding anything that is a reminder of the miscarriage; and persistent edginess or distress or both. Can manifest within hours of the event. Lasts no longer than four weeks.

adenomyosis. Like endometriosis, this condition involves small amounts of uterine lining growing inside the uterine muscle. Can cause heavy, painful periods and an elevated risk of miscarriage.

adjustment disorder. Experiencing more stress than would normally be expected in response to a pregnancy loss, to the point where it causes significant problems in your life. Symptoms start within three months of the loss and last no longer than six months after the loss.

amniocentesis. Procedure in which amniotic fluid is removed from the uterus for testing or treatment.

anembryonic pregnancy. When an early embryo never develops or when it stops developing, is resorbed, and leaves an empty gestational sac. The reason this occurs is often unknown, but it may be due to chromosomal abnormalities in the fertilized egg. Also called a blighted ovum.

anti-inflammatories. Group of pain medications that include ibuprofen, naproxen sodium and acetaminophen. The best pain medication for the cramps associated with your period or a miscarriage. Also good for treating headaches and fevers.

assisted reproductive technology. Procedures used to help with fertility or prevent genetic problems and assist with the conception of a child. In vitro fertilization (IVF) is the most effective form of assisted reproductive technology.

bicornuate uterus. Condition present from birth in which the uterus has two cavities instead of one. Can increase the risk of miscarriage or premature birth.

buccal administration. Taking medication by placing it in the mouth, between the cheek and gums, and letting it dissolve there.

cervical balloon. Small, inflatable balloon at the end of a tube that can be placed through the cervix to open (dilate) it.

cervical insufficiency. Painless opening (dilation) of the cervix. Sometimes can be treated with a procedure to stitch the cervix closed (cerclage) but may lead to pregnancy loss. Also called cervical incompetence.

cervix. The opening to the womb (uterus) at the inside end of the vagina. Needs to open (dilate) to allow delivery of a baby and placenta.

chemical pregnancy. A pregnancy that hasn't progressed far enough to create tissue visible on an ultrasound. In these pregnancies, the egg and sperm joined and the resulting embryo implanted and started making pregnancy hormones, but the pregnancy rapidly stopped developing.

choriocarcinoma. Abnormal growth of the placenta that can continue to grow even after a procedure to remove it. Most often happens after a complete molar pregnancy. Can become cancerous by spreading to other organs.

chorionic villus sampling (CVS). Procedure that removes a small sample of a growing placenta (chorionic villi) where it joins the uterus. Involves placing a long, skinny needle through the cervix or through the belly, using ultrasound as a guide. Used to test for chromosomal abnormalities.

complete miscarriage. When the body has passed all of the pregnancy tissue out of the uterus. May also be called a spontaneous abortion.

complete molar pregnancy. A pregnancy that contains only placental tissue and no embryo or fetus. Can lead to pregnancy tissue spreading throughout the body.

complicated (prolonged) grief. Long-lasting and severe painful emotions that make it difficult to recover from a loss. Feelings of grief linger or get worse instead of fading or resolving.

conscious sedation. Type of anesthesia that reduces pain and helps you relax, but leaves you awake. Often involves two medications, fentanyl and midazolam. May leave you feeling drowsy the rest of the day. Also called IV sedation.

crown-rump length. Measurement from the top of a baby's head to the baby's bum, taken from the side when the baby is curled up in the shape of a comma.

didelphys. Rare birth defect in which a person is born with a double uterus. Can increase the risk of miscarriage or premature birth.

Dilapan. Type of cervical dilator. Works to open the cervix by swelling in size like a sponge, absorbing water, and causing the cervix to release hormones that trigger it to soften and dilate.

dilation and curettage (D&C). Two-step procedure of stretching open the natural opening of your cervix with dilators, then removing all of the pregnancy tissue, typically with suction rather than scraping with a metal instrument (curetting). Performed in the first trimester of pregnancy. Also called vacuum or suction aspiration. Sometimes called suction curettage.

dilation and evacuation (D&E). Two-step process of opening (dilating) the cervix with medication or cervical dilators (or both) and evacuating or removing a pregnancy and placenta. Performed in the second trimester of pregnancy.

Doppler monitor. Hand-held wand that uses ultrasound waves to detect the fetal heartbeat. Used at every prenatal visit after about 12 weeks of pregnancy to make sure the heartbeat sounds normal. Also a circular paddle that attaches to a stretchy band around your belly when you're being monitored for a longer period of time.

eclampsia. Essentially, preeclampsia with seizures. Develops when preeclampsia isn't controlled.

ectopic pregnancy. A pregnancy growing outside of the uterine cavity. Can be in the fallopian tubes, the cervix, the corners of the uterus, a cesarean section scar, an ovary or anywhere in the belly.

electric vacuum aspiration. Use of an electric vacuum pump to remove pregnancy tissue from the uterus. Noisier than a manual vacuum. Most often used in a procedure or operating room, though can also be used in a doctor's office.

embolization. Minor procedure during which a radiologist uses a slender, flexible tube (catheter) to inject small particles (embolic agents) into arteries to decreases blood flow and blocks blood vessels. Used to control excessive bleeding after dilation and curettage (D&C) or dilation and evacuation (D&E).

embryo. A baby in the earliest stage of development. Lasts from shortly after fertilization of the egg by the sperm until eight weeks after conception (10 weeks of pregnancy).

embryonic demise. An embryo has formed but stops developing and dies before any symptoms of pregnancy loss occur.

endometriosis. Condition in which tissue similar to the lining of the uterus grows outside of the uterus on other tissues and organs, most often on the lining of the pelvis, ovaries (where it can cause cysts), fallopian tubes and ligaments that hold the uterus in place. Diagnosis can only be confirmed officially during surgery (usually laparoscopy), when visible implants can be removed. Symptoms of pelvic pain can be managed with hormonal birth control and anti-inflammatories. One of the leading causes of chronic pelvic pain in women.

epidural anesthesia. Use of a catheter placed in the back to deliver numbing medication (anesthetic) to the spinal column. Reduces or eliminates pain during labor.

episiotomy. Incision made in the tissue between the vaginal opening and the anus (perineum) during childbirth. Widens the opening to make it easier for a baby to deliver.

expectant management. Process of waiting for a miscarriage to begin naturally, without medication or a procedure. Also known as waiting it out.

fallopian tubes. Pair of tubes that eggs travel through to get from the ovaries to the uterus. Each month, during a process called ovulation, one of the ovaries releases an egg that travels down one of the fallopian tubes, where it may or may not be fertilized by a sperm.

fetal demise. The fetus stops developing and dies before any symptoms of pregnancy loss occur.

fetus. Baby inside the uterus after the first 10 weeks of pregnancy.

fibroids. Growths in the uterus made of muscle and fibrous tissue. Can be embedded in the wall of the uterus, stick out from the uterus like mouse ears or (the kind that may be linked to miscarriage) extend into the uterine cavity. Can cause heavy or painful periods, which can be managed with medication. Can be removed with surgery in some cases. Sometimes referred to as noncancerous (benign) tumors, leiomyomas (lie-o-my-O-muhs) or myomas.

general anesthesia. The use of a combination of medications that put you in a sleep-like state before a surgery or other medical procedure.

generalized anxiety disorder. Persistent, excessive, intrusive worry that occurs on most days and last for more than six months.

gestational sac. Membrane that surrounds fluid and a growing pregnancy. Also called the pregnancy sac.

gestational trophoblastic disease. Another term for a molar pregnancy.

HELLP syndrome. Stands for hemolysis (the destruction of red blood cells), elevated liver enzymes and low platelets. A more severe form of preeclampsia, which can quickly become life-threatening for both the baby and the pregnant person.

human chorionic gonadotropin (HCG). Hormone found in the blood and urine of someone who's pregnant. Very high levels of this hormone may indicate a molar pregnancy. May also be referred to as beta-HCG or simply beta.

hydatidiform mole. Another term for a molar pregnancy.

hysterosalpingogram (HSG). Radiology procedure used to look at the uterus and fallopian tubes. Involves placing a catheter into the cervix, injecting dye and taking X-rays of the pelvis.

hysteroscopy. Procedure that involves placing a camera into the uterus through the vagina and cervix and then filling the uterus with fluid. Allows doctors to remove polyps and fibroids that might be causing heavy or irregular bleeding or causing miscarriages.

incomplete abortion. When the uterus has contracted and passed out some but not all of the pregnancy tissue.

induction. Process of starting labor contractions with medications. Makes the cervix open so the baby and placenta can be delivered.

inevitable abortion. When the cervix is dilated (open) and pregnancy tissue will soon pass out of the uterus.

inpatient. Hospital visit that requires an overnight stay.

intrauterine growth restriction. Condition in which a baby isn't growing as much as he or she should be. Specifically, this is when the estimated fetal weight is below the 10th percentile for the baby's gestational age.

intravenous (IV). When a tiny, plastic tube (catheter) is placed into a vein in your hand or your arm. Allows a nurse or doctor to give fluids and medications.

invasive mole. When tissue from a molar pregnancy penetrates deep into the middle layer of the uterine wall and causes heavy vaginal bleeding.

labor and delivery (L&D). Unit in a hospital where people go through the process of labor and delivery of a baby.

laminaria. Most common form of cervical dilator. About the size of matchsticks and made of seaweed, laminaria open the cervix by swelling in size like a sponge, absorbing water, and causing the cervix to release hormones that trigger it to soften and dilate.

laparoscopy. When a surgeon makes a series of small (5 to 10 mm) incisions in your belly button and on your abdomen to perform procedures guided by a camera. Done while you're completely asleep (under general anesthesia). Often referred to as having a scope. Usually doesn't require an overnight hospital stay.

last menstrual period (LMP). Refers to the date of the first day of bleeding of your last normal period. Can be recorded on a calendar or in an app as the first day you needed to use menstrual protection that cycle.

lidocaine. Local anesthesic (numbing medication). Injected around the cervix during a procedure, particularly for the treatment of a miscarriage.

local anesthesia. Injection of a numbing medication into an area prior to a procedure to reduce pain. Injected into the vagina around the cervix during a D&C for a miscarriage.

magnetic resonance imaging (MRI). Uses a magnetic field and radio waves to create cross-sectional images of the head and body. Can create detailed images of the inside of the uterus if a structural problem is suspected. Can also be used to detail the anatomy of the fetus if an abnormality is seen with ultrasound.

manual vacuum aspiration (MVA). Use of a hand-held, hand-activated large plastic syringe to remove pregnancy tissue from the uterus. Can be used for a procedure in a doctor's office or in the emergency room.

maternal-fetal medicine (MFM). Subspecialty of obstetrics concerned with the obstetric, medical, genetic and surgical complications of pregnancy and their effects on pregnant people and fetuses. You may see an MFM specialist before pregnancy if you have a chronic medical condition or have had multiple pregnancy losses. Or you may see an MFM specialist during pregnancy if you or the baby develops a complication.

medical management. Using a regimen of medications to complete your miscarriage by inducing bleeding and cramping.

methotrexate. Medication that stops the growth of cells that are rapidly dividing, such as pregnancy cells. Given as an injection into a muscle, its use requires careful monitoring.

methylergonovine. Medication used to prevent and control bleeding from the uterus that can happen after childbirth or a miscarriage.

mifepristone. Medication sometimes used in the medical treatment of miscarriages. Taken as a single pill in a doctor's office. Not currently available by prescription. Often called "mife" (pronounced MIF-ee) for short.

miscarriage. Natural end, death or loss of a pregnancy. Traditionally refers to a first trimester spontaneous loss of a pregnancy inside the uterus.

misoprostol. Medication almost always used in the medical treatment of miscarriage. Taken as multiple pills, it's swallowed, tucked into your cheeks (buccally) or placed in the vagina. Available by prescription, but not always immediately available at the pharmacy. Often called "miso" for short.

missed abortion. When a pregnancy has stopped developing but the uterus hasn't begun to expel the pregnancy tissue hasn't yet begun.

moderate sedation. Type of anesthesia that elicits feelings of relaxation and drowsiness, given before a medical procedure. You may feel movement or pressure during the procedure, but you shouldn't feel severe pain. Also called IV or conscious sedation.

molar pregnancy. Rare type of pregnancy complication in which the cells that typically develop into the placenta don't develop as they should. There are two types: complete molar pregnancy and partial molar pregnancy. Also known as hydatidiform mole.

multifetal pregnancy reduction. Process of reducing one or more fetuses in a multiple gestation (triplets, quadruplets). Improves the chances that the remaining fetuses will be born healthy.

nonsteroidal anti-inflammatory drugs (NSAIDs). Medications commonly used to treat pain and inflammation. Can't be taken during pregnancy but are often used in the treatment of miscarriage and pregnancy loss. Include ibuprofen and naproxen sodium.

outpatient. Hospital visit that doesn't require an overnight stay.

ovaries. Part of the female reproductive system. There are two ovaries, one on each side of the uterus. Ovaries produce eggs (ova) and the hormones estrogen and progesterone. Eggs travel from the ovaries into the fallopian tubes; this is where fertilization with sperm takes place and a pregnancy begins.

ovulation. Release of an egg from an ovary. Fertilization must occur within about 24 hours of ovulation if pregnancy is to happen.

oxytocin. Medication that causes the cervix to open (dilate) and the uterus to contract, starting the labor process. Given in a slow drip through a thin tube that's placed in a vein in the arm or hand (IV). Also called Pitocin, or Pit for short.

paracervical block. Injection of a numbing medication (anesthetic) through the wall of the vagina around the cervix. Causes a cramping sensation when the medication goes in. Doesn't take away all of the pain but makes the procedure more comfortable.

partial molar pregnancy. A pregnancy complication in which the embryo has too many chromosomes, which can't lead to the growth of a healthy baby. The embryo or fetus won't live to be born. Also called an incomplete mole.

pelvic inflammatory disease (PID). Treatable with antibiotics, this infection may cause fever, nausea and pelvic pain. Can cause scarring in your pelvis that can affect your fallopian tubes and make it difficult for sperm to reach an egg. Most often, caused by a sexually transmitted infection, like chlamydia or gonorrhea, that moves up from the cervix into the uterus and spreads throughout the pelvis. Sometimes may be caused by normal vaginal bacteria.

perforation. Incredibly rare complication of a D&C in which an instrument makes a small hole in the wall of the uterus. May be managed by watching you as you heal in the hospital or with a follow-up visit. In some cases requires an additional surgery to make sure there is no injury to other organs in the pelvis.

persistent gestational trophoblastic neoplasia. Any tissue from a molar pregnancy that remains and continues to grow after a dilation and curettage (D&C).

placental abruption. Uncommon, serious complication of pregnancy that occurs when the placenta partly or completely separates from the inner wall of the uterus before delivery. Can decrease or block the baby's supply of oxygen and nutrients and cause heavy bleeding in the pregnant person.

postpartum depression. Feelings of extreme sadness, anxiety and exhaustion that make it difficult for a people to care for themselves or others or to go through daily life. Often accompanied by feelings of guilt or hopelessness. Can occur during a pregnancy or up to a year after giving birth or having a loss.

post-traumatic stress disorder. Mental health condition triggered by experiencing or witnessing a terrifying event. Symptoms may include flashbacks, nightmares and severe anxiety, as well as uncontrollable thoughts about the event. May start within one month of a traumatic event, but sometimes symptoms may not appear until years afterward. Symptoms cause significant problems in social or work situations and in relationships. They can also interfere with the ability to go about normal daily tasks.

preeclampsia. Pregnancy complication characterized by high blood pressure and signs of damage to another organ system, most often the liver or kidneys. Usually begins after 20 weeks of pregnancy in someone whose blood pressure had been within the standard range. Left untreated, preeclampsia can lead to serious — even fatal — complications for both the pregnant person and the baby.

pregnancy of unknown location. When you have a positive pregnancy test but your doctor can't see the pregnancy on an ultrasound.

pregnancy sac. Membrane that surrounds fluid and a growing pregnancy. Also called the gestational sac.

pre-implantation testing. Test that may be used when attempting to conceive a child through in vitro fertilization. Also called pre-implantation genetic diagnosis.

preterm prelabor rupture of membranes (PPROM). When the "bag of water" inside the uterus that holds the baby develops a tear, also known as breaking your water. This allows the amniotic fluid surrounding the baby to escape and infection to develop. Happens if your water breaks before the 37th week of pregnancy.

radiofrequency ablation. Method of reducing a pregnancy with multiple fetuses. Uses a small needle device to send electric currents to interrupt the blood flow from the umbilical cord to one or more fetuses.

recurrent pregnancy loss. Two or more failed pregnancies in a row. The definition of *loss* can include pregnancies that were confirmed with a pregnancy test or with an ultrasound.

reproductive endocrinologist (REI). Subspecialty of OB-GYN that focuses on diagnosing and treating conditions that can stop conception and make it difficult for a person to carry a pregnancy to term. You may see an REI if you're experiencing recurrent pregnancy loss.

retained placenta. When part or all of the placenta doesn't deliver after the baby. Sometimes the placenta can be removed with the doctor's hand, but in the second trimester, it often needs a vacuum aspiration.

Rh_0(D) immune globulin (Rhogam). Medication used to prevent Rh immunization, where a person with Rh-negative blood develops antibodies after exposure to Rh-positive blood. Given to any Rh-negative pregnant person after bleeding in pregnancy, after treatment of an ectopic pregnancy or after delivery of a baby.

sac diameter. Measurement of a pregnancy (gestational) sac. Often, an ultrasound technician measures the length, width and height of the sac, then takes the average of the measurements to find the mean (average) sac diameter, which can be used to calculate how far along a pregnancy is.

selective reduction. Process of reducing one or more fetuses in a multiple gestation (triplets, quadruplets). Performed when one fetus has an anomaly, or when a medical condition threatens the lives of one or more fetuses. Improves the chances that the remaining fetuses will be born healthy.

sonohysterogram. Ultrasound procedure used to look at the cavity of the uterus. Involves placing a catheter into the cervix, injecting salt water (saline) and performing an ultrasound of the uterus. Also known as a saline infusion sonogram or SIS.

speculum. Plastic or metal hinged instrument shaped like a duck's bill that's used to spread open the vaginal walls so a doctor can see the vagina and the cervix.

spontaneous abortion. When the body has passed all of the pregnancy tissue without medication or a procedure. Also called a miscarriage.

stillbirth. When a baby dies in the womb (*in utero*, meaning in the uterus) after 20 weeks of pregnancy.

surgical management. Using a procedure to complete a miscarriage. Also often referred to as a dilation and curettage (D&C).

therapeutic abortion. Abortion performed to save the life or health (physical or mental) of a pregnant person.

threatened abortion. When bleeding or cramping is happening, but the cervix hasn't opened (dilated). An ultrasound shows no signs of trouble with the pregnancy.

transvaginal ultrasound. Used most often during early pregnancy and when a transabdominal ultrasound doesn't provide enough information. A wandlike device called a transducer is placed in the vagina. It sends out sound waves, gathers the reflections and turns them into a grainy 2D image.

trimester. Three-month period of pregnancy. First trimester roughly corresponds to the first three months, and so on.

tubal pregnancy. A pregnancy in the fallopian tube between the ovary and the uterus. Most common ectopic pregnancy location.

ultrasound. Imaging technique that uses sound waves to produce images of a pregnancy in the uterus. Fetal ultrasound images can help your doctor evaluate your baby's growth and development and monitor your pregnancy. In some cases, fetal ultrasound is used to evaluate possible problems or help confirm a diagnosis. May be performed on your belly (transabdominal) or with a wandlike device (transducer) placed in your vagina (transvaginal).

unicornuate uterus. Rare genetic condition in which only half of the uterus forms. Smaller than a typical uterus and has only one fallopian tube. Can make it difficult to carry a pregnancy to term.

uterine septum. Abnormality of the uterus present since birth, this muscular and fibrous band of tissue extends from the top of the uterine cavity down into the middle of the cavity, dividing the uterine cavity into two sections. This septum may be thin or thick, and it can often be removed with surgery.

uterus. The organ inside of which an unborn baby develops. Also called a womb.

vacuum aspiration. Another name for a dilation and curettage (D&C) procedure. Removes the contents of the uterus through a plastic or metal cannula attached to a vacuum source.

viability. The ability to continue to grow and develop. In pregnancy, usually refers to the ability of a baby to survive outside the womb. Influenced by the age of the pregnancy along with the size and health of the baby. The threshold of viability is the point in the pregnancy where the baby can live outside of your body, with or without medical help. Generally, it's 23 or 24 weeks of pregnancy, but at the most-advanced hospitals, it can be as early as 22 weeks.

viable pregnancy. A pregnancy that appears to be healthy. The embryo is visible in the uterus, and if it's large enough, it has a heartbeat.

yolk sac. Provides nutrition and blood cells to a developing embryo before the placenta is formed and can take over. Also helps form the umbilical cord. Important in early pregnancy because it's a marker of how healthy the pregnancy is and where it's located.

Index

R

radiofrequency ablation, 216, 228

recurrent losses
about, 35, 151–153
anatomical abnormalities and,
154–157
causes of, 154–162
genetic abnormalities and, 154,
159–162
hormonal imbalances and, 154,
158–159
immune conditions and, 154,
157–158
next pregnancy and, 163–164
questions to ask, 165
testing and, 153–154, 156–161, 162
treatment and, 157, 158, 159, 161–162

relief, 243

remembrance of loss
about, 313–314
burial and, 322–323
ceremonies, 320–321
customs for, 321
donations in, 323
first trimester loss and, 314, 318
memory box and, 315, 316, 319
naming the baby and, 318–319
ongoing, 324–325
self-reflection and, 326-327

renal agenesis, 221

retained tissue, 103–104

S

sadness, 266–267, 272
See also depression

same-sex couples, 294

secondary infertility, 161

second trimester pregnancy loss
baby abnormalities and, 111
baby heartbeat and, 114
bleeding and cramping and, 113
causes of, 110–112
expectant management and,
115–116
follow-up with doctor, 128–129
getting pregnant again and, 330,
336

labor induction and, 115, 116,
117–119
questions to ask, 130–131
treatment options, 114–128
warning signs, 113–114
See also dilation and curettage
(D&C)

selective reduction, 216, 225–227

sex and miscarriages, 21, 252–254, 332

sex and pregnancy, 293

spina bifida, 220

spontaneous abortion, 42, 44

spotting, 173–174

stigma, reducing, 346–349

stillbirth
about, 133–134
causes of, 136–137, 146–147
C-section and, 143, 334
defined, 135
diagnosis of, 138–145
expectant management and, 139
fetal conditions and, 138
follow-up with doctor, 145–146
getting pregnant again and,
329–330
labor induction and, 139, 140–145
questions to ask, 148–149
recovery, 144–145
risk factors, 134

structural fetal abnormalities, 221

support, asking for, 310

support groups and counseling,
282–283

support network, 308–309

surgical management
about, 91
bleeding and cramping and,
100–103, 104
defined, 48
medications before, 93
in an office, 97–98
in an operating room, 98–99
option comparison, 60–61
questions to ask, 106–107
risks of, 51
steps for, 94–97
support person during, 99
in a surgical suite, 98
when it's over, 100–105

Acknowledgments

Writing is simultaneously one of the hardest and one of the most rewarding things I've ever pursued. (Just like parenthood, come to think of it.) Completing this book allowed my second deepest dream to come true. But publishing a book is the intellectual equivalent of the cycling teams in the Tour de France — team leaders earn the prize, but they would never be able to cross the finish line without the support of their teammates.

To the team at Mayo Clinic Press, thank you for believing in this book and giving me the gentlest introduction possible to the world of publishing. Stephanie Vaughan is the editor of my dreams. She got to know me as a person as well as a writer and understood what I wanted this book to express on every level. Working with her was never work. Thank you for making me sound like the doctor I strive to be.

Jay Koski's art direction brought my vision for this book into reality. Gunnar Soroos crafted a template that is somehow both clean and warm. Matt Meyer made medical equipment look much less scary and made memory items even more inviting. Amanda Knapp made all the irregular pieces of my writing fit into a coherent whole. Mike Nienow risked vision loss by scouring countless ultrasounds until he found just the right images. The careful proofing by Miranda Attlesey, Donna Hanson, Nancy Jacoby and Julie Maas outstrip even my attention to detail and soothed my compulsive soul. Dr. Mari Charisse Trinidad and Julie Lamppa gave thoughtful comments during their review that fortified the foundation of the book. Dan Harke and Nina Wiener, in the middle of a pandemic, saw the promise of this book and adopted me into the Mayo Clinic Press stable. And to everyone else on the Mayo Clinic Press team who helped to midwife this book into existence, thank you for getting us safely through the delivery.

To Rita Rosenkranz, my intrepid agent — thank you for believing in me and this book and for taking a chance on a first-time author.

To Lisa Tener, the coach I met at a Boston leadership course, who confirmed that I had a promising idea for a book. Thank you for your words of wisdom and encouragement.

To Jody Rein and Michael Larsen, whose guide to writing book proposals meant I didn't need to self-publish. Your book is a service to every aspiring author.

To my first readers, Lorraine Ash, Molly Finneseth, Sherokee Ilse, Dr. Aviva-Lee Parritz, Dr. Beri Ridgeway and Dr. Kathy Sharpless. The book is immeasurably better because of the time you took to read early manuscripts and offer me thoughtful feedback. To Dr. Steve Fiascone, thank you for reviewing the most complicated chapter of the book.

To Kayla Voigt, the best listener I know. Thank you for getting the thoughts in my head onto paper. Your questions and insights turned a rocky first draft into something resembling an actual book. I couldn't have done this without you.

To Dr. Sree Gaddipati, who saved my life, and Dr. Mike Plevyak. Thank you for getting me safely through my pregnancies.

To my mental health team, Andrea Jewel, Maggie Leblanc and Julie Rosen, who made me whole when I was feeling most broken.

To my dearest friends Paula Castaño (92%), Serena Chao (BMC x2 bestie) and Kerrin Flanagan (*vive le vent*). You make me feel seen, keep me grounded and always make me feel loved.

To my patients. You let me into your lives and shared with me your most honest moments. I hope I taught you half as much as you taught me.

To my mother, Christine O'Connell. You introduced me to books from toddlerhood and encouraged my love of reading, even when it meant making constant trips to the public library and raiding your own bookshelves. You have been the wind beneath my wings my entire life, and you've believed that there's nothing I couldn't do. I'm the writer/doctor/mother/woman I am because of you.

To Ben, who introduced me to (step)motherhood. Marrying your dad meant that I got to be a mom — you're my free gift with purchase. You made it easy for me from the start, and I've been so proud watching you grow.

To Zachary and Dexter. You're my treasures at the end of the mission, the Peach for my Mario. You make the journey worth it, and I can't imagine my life without either of you. I'm so proud to be your mom, and I love you to the end of the universe and back. We are totally in the good place.

And to my stalwart partner, Chad. Thank you for your loving encouragement, your crack copyediting, and your constant support of my late nights and weekends holed up in my cloffice. We've handled more than our fair share of crises — our marriage has been forged in the fire, and we've come out stronger on the other side. You put your arms around me and I'm home. I can't wait to see what the journey still holds in store for us.

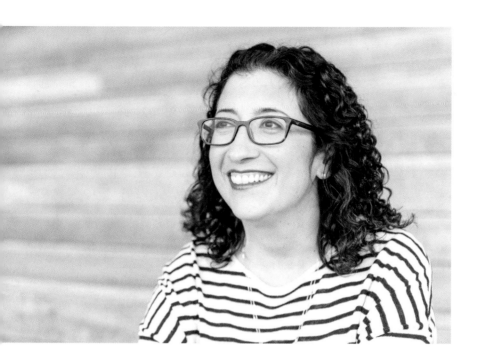

Kate White, M.D., M.P.H., is an associate professor of obstetrics and gynecology at the Boston University School of Medicine, and the vice chair of academics in the OB-GYN department at Boston Medical Center. She is a fellow of the American College of Obstetricians and Gynecologists and of the Society of Family Planning, and a member of the American Public Health Association.

A board-certified OB-GYN, Dr. Kate has been caring for patients for more than 20 years, helping them navigate periods, childbirth, pregnancy loss and every other stage leading up to menopause. She also conducts research in contraception, has been continuously grant funded for 15 years, and frequently lectures regionally and nationally on topics related to reproductive health. Dr. Kate lives outside of Boston with her husband and their three children.

Read Dr. Kate's firsthand, in-depth account of experiencing and healing after pregnancy loss with her daughter, Samantha, in *Glamour* magazine at *www.glamour.com/story/recovering-after-a-miscarriage-the-baby-i-lost-and-the-life-she-gave-me.*